Rustic Healthy

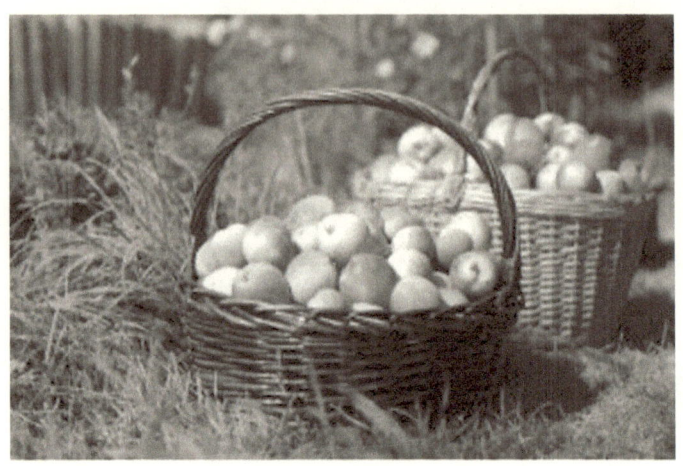

On the Cover

The Rustic Apple

The rustic *organic* apple that is, and it's constituents, *organic* apple juice and raw apple cider vinegar (one of my personal healthy favorites) have a multitude of benefits it seems, so I chose to feature the rustic *organic* basket of apples "on the cover". Just a few health benefits of the apple? . . . fights plaque so you get whiter, healthier teeth, helps avoid Alzheimer's (caused by plaque also?), protects against Parkinson's, curbs all sorts of cancers, (liver cancer, breast cancer, stomach cancer) decreases your risk of diabetes, reduces cholesterol! Get a healthier heart reducing plaque (again) and preventing hardening of the arteries (by reducing plaque!). Prevents gallstones, controls your weight and cholesterol levels. Beats diarrhea and constipation both. Averts hemorrhoids. Detoxifies your liver (one of the best and easiest ways to do this *and very* important to do). Prevents cataracts, (being rich in antioxidants), and apples having quercetin can help boost and fortify your immune system!

Therefore . . . it may very well be true? . . .

"An apple a day keeps the doctor away" afterall! . . .

An *organic* apple, that is :)

In *rustic health,*

rustichealthy :)

Rustic Healthy

How to get healthy, be happy (*and* lose some weight?) without really trying :)

RusticHealthy

Rev. date: 06/17/2013

To order additional copies of this book, contact:
Xlibris
1-888-795-4274
www.Xlibris.com
Orders@Xlibris.com
130756

Contents

Chapter 1: Get Healthy, Be Happy 7

Chapter 2: It's Not Just About Me 16

Chapter 3: Go Organic Or 24

Chapter 4: It Takes Time 32

Chapter 5: What do we get? 41

Chapter 6: How to Easily Detox 55

Chapter 7: Just Say No To GMO and CAFO 61

Chapter 8: Consider the Cost 67

Chapter 9: Drink Water 72

Chapter 10: On To Exercise! 75

Chapter 11: My First 'Alternative' Experience 78

Chapter 12: It's a "LivingStyle" 80

Chapter 13: My Own Happy Conclusion 90

Rustic's Healthy Commentaries

Rustic Commentary 1: My Hypothyroidism 97

Rustic Commentary 2: The Newest "Scape Goat" 102

Rustic Commentary 3: Whose Guinea Pig are You? 104

Rustic Commentary 4: Bad Medicine:/ in the "Belly of the Beast"

and the "Dose of the Vitamin" 106

Rustic Commentary 5: "Liar, Fraud!" 111

Rustic Commentary 6: Why Do My Placebos Work? 115

Rustic Commentary 7: Vegan/Vegetarian or Organic Omnivore 117

Rustic Commentary 8: What's the Harm Rethink 120

Rustic Commentary 9: The Belly of the Beast

and "Green Coffee Beans" 123

Rustic Commentary 10: Pain (Headache and Heartburn) Management ... 127

Rustic Commentary 11: Anecdotal vs. Clinical........................ 131

Rustic Commentary 12: Vitamins :) vs. Vaccines :/ 135

Rustic Commentary 13: Nip it in the Bud! 139

Rustic Commentary 14: Barking up the Wrong Tree (again)...... 142

Rustic Commentary 15: Vitamin C (with Bioflavanoids & Rosehips)

Still my Stealth Fav :) 145

Rustic Commentary 16: From Fluoride to Freedom:) 151

Rustic Commentary 17: On the Cold War Front 156

Rustic Commentary 18: Dealing with "death trolls" 160

Rustic Commentary 19: A few Thank you's very much Appreciated 166

Rustic Healthy 20: On Defending Omnivores (taking on the Vegans :) ... 168

Rustic Commentary 21: The New Snake Oil 175

Rustic Healthy "Anecdotal" Testimonials

"Let Food be thy Medicine . . ."... 178

Rustic's Healthy Recipes :) 187

Chapter 1

Get *Healthy*, Be Happy

My Message Here and How it Began

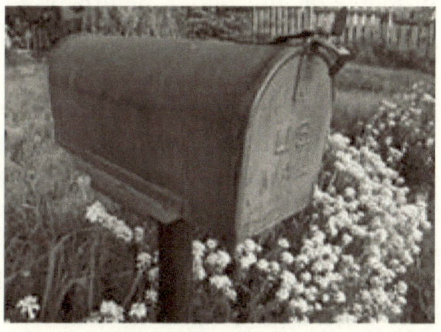

The fellow who has not had any experience is so dumb he doesn't know a thing can't be done, and he goes ahead and does it. Charles F. Kettering

My message here is a *simple* one actually (hence "Rustic"), regarding health (hence "Healthy":) and how you, and just about anyone you may know could, and *should* have much better *healthcare* (and perhaps learn how *affordable* it can be afterall?!). However, it has nothing to do with *"healthcare"* as in the media. And, it has little to do with any conventional or popular dieting and weight loss or fitness programs (though many are healthy and many on them are happy). Not putting down anyone's healthy fitness and weightloss program! However "Rustic Healthy" is not a diet! But *if you are happy* with the diet or fitness program you're on you just might receive a little help, and perhaps learn a few other things from here too about health (it is my hope anyway). If you are *happy* with the diet or fitness program you're on you may also receive a little help, and perhaps learn a few other things from here too (it is my hope anyway). Actually it's more about getting healthy from whatever age, stage or condition you're in . . . "Even stage 4 cancer??" . . . hmmm well, we shall see. Now, I've been informed that I am "cruel beyond belief" presenting anything hopeful in that case to *anyone*, but, I'm going to let the reader decide for themselves. *Obviously* I cannot *guarantee* any such thing. But I do believe they are great to hear about and believe one would want to know them, and have some very possible good options even at that stage? (I would like to know them for myself anyway). As I stated in the "Book Summary" I *am not* a doctor, health professional, or nutritionist for that matter. So the following is according to me, my own unprofessional, non-clinical studied "anecdotal" experience (as well as some others I've come across) and what I've encountered (and think I've learned :) hoping you will carefully look into these things for *yourself* before accepting or rejecting anything I'm presenting here, or what anyone else says about them too. Please, always check with your own doctor or alternative health professional if something may or may not be right for you as well!

Personally my experience has been more with respiratory problems (though I do have others as you will well see:). I've had to deal with bronchitis since a child (my parents being told to consider moving to Arizona) and pretty bad asthma as an adult (being on 4 asthma medications including 2 inhalers, and steroids) and now without any use of conventional meds for over 4 years now, thus, the "get healthy" part! Being on (and off:) diets most of my life, it's been a long downward battle. Yes I said *downward*, because I never did find a way to conquer it with any diet that I've tried anyway :p (though I know many have done so amazingly, and I give *a lot* of credit to!). This isn't that kind of testimony. It's the testimony of how I've come to learn a few things only, not even considering losing weight any longer, totally giving up (fed up actually:) to find what was the stumbling block to any effort I've made. I am not talking about a trick, or formula in a pill, but it actually is *better* (I believe anyway). It has little or nothing to do with "discipline", "strong will", counting, weighing, etc. And you'll perhaps see truly once and for all time how it never was *your* fault to begin with. You'll actually be able to live very happy with it, and perhaps return to "normal" regarding food and *diet* as well, if you've been battling for years as I have. I want to *lift* the weight off your shoulders rather. Thus, the "be happy" part.

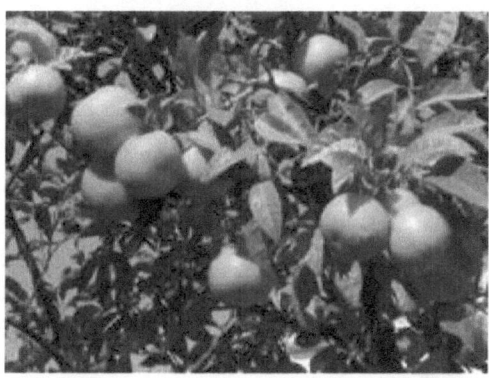

It began with Vitamin C! an *awesome* vitamin for allergies and a natural antihistamine (among other things so I'm finding out) which did indeed help my asthma! However, you should know (as I am told as well, many times in 'health' forums) that this is "not possible" because . . . "clinical studies" do not show it, and health alternative studies that *do* show it (of which I have found quite a few actually) do not prove it. That it's a "placebo" (please see my commentary on "Why My Placebos Work":). I've also been told I *didn't have* asthma (?) or I *didn't know* I didn't have asthma (!) or the doctors didn't know I didn't have asthma(?!) but put me on 4 asthma meds anyway hmmmm :) Another was, I did but it "comes and goes" at will and nothing I did or took helped . . . In any case! it did help for years (according to me anyway, and I'm the one writing this book afterall:) however it was not enough to *keep* attacks away so I found (according to me too).

Ok so with that out of the way :), to the best that I can describe anyway, in the beginning of an attack, I would take usually 500 mg to 1000 mg vitamin C supplement, wait a few minutes and it would many times subside. Why I thought of Vitamin C to take at the time was I had heard it helps with colds (though I've been told I'm wrong about that too) and allergies "Vitamin C for allergy", (of course I'm wrong about that also:) so perhaps it would help with other respiratory conditions such as mine (whatever it was)? If it didn't *naturally* I would take my inhaler. I'm not suggesting *anyone not* take their inhaler or medicine if they need it. Please keep it right there with you. I still have an inhaler myself (just rarely need to use it now). I also began realizing I needed something for infections because that's when I noticed my asthma would act up at times also and Vitamin C alone was not doing it all the time. I remembered (from perhaps my mom reading about vitamins) "Vitamin A for infection", and so looked for Vitamin A (beta carotene) supplements, and somehow, can't say exactly why at the time, but I thought of fish oil (perhaps remembering 'cod liver oil as a child), and added that as well, which did seem to have a better effect!

Sometimes with Vit C alone I would still have a "tightening" when breathing the best I can describe it but when I added the Vit A and fish oil it "opened" or "loosened" a little easier. I do believe everyone is different, but those are some basics that I have and still use. However it was not on a daily basis then (not thinking in terms of strengthening and *prevention* which happens to be very important to me now). Actually, my asthma acted up not only when I had an infection but during allergy season (four years ago it was because of an awful "mold" condition here in rural Virginia), and then when I had a cold, or when I was stressed, or when in a polluted environment (maybe a smoking area or subway station when I worked in NYC), or when I over exerted myself (running for a bus), or the weather was bad. Pretty much . . . it could happen anytime. I now take 1000 mg Vit. C every day which I believe now helps *prevent* my attacks to begin with (more if I need it, if I feel I'm coming down with something, and for me it's usually in the colder weather also). I'll use things like apple cider vinegar now (a natural anti-viral), organic honey (a natural anti-bacterial) and cinnamon also (a natural anti-biotic). If you look up the health benefits of any of those you would be absolutely *amazed* at the multi benefits reaped as well! An all natural (organic preferably) powdered fruit and vegetable source for Vitamin C such as kamu kamu berry (a high source of Vitamin C) is great too.

Other benefits of Vitamin C?

What's absolutely amazing about all the vitamins and nutrients and natural foods also (like honey, cinnamon and apple cider vinegar) is, the more I learn about them? the *more benefits* they seem to produce! So here are some other amazing benefits of Vitamin C:

> **promotes healing of all body cells**
> **essential for building collagen** (less wrinkles? yes!)
> **helps prevent cancer and heart disease!**
> **detoxifies the body** (absolutely need this)
> **supports the good bacteria in your gut**
> **kills candida, bacteria, fungi, viruses** (colds, flu?), **and parasites**
> **prevents hardening of the arteries** (that's always a good thing:)
> **neutralizes harmful environmental and bacterial toxins**
> **protects us from pollution and dangerous pesticides**
> **destroys free radicals** (a real warrior)
> **combats stress** (cool!)

acts as an antidepressant (nice, maybe what more need)
removes heavy metals like mercury and lead
lowers high cholesterol (super!)
a natural antihistamine (for allergies)

*　　*　　*

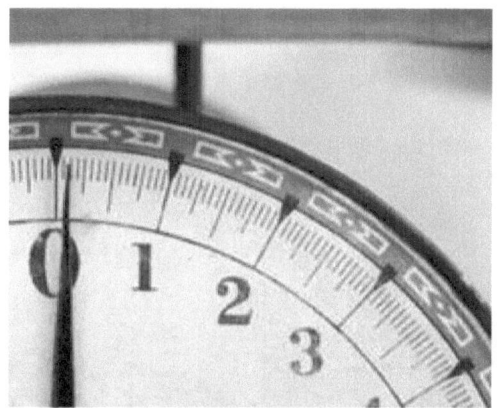

My weight problem started after I quit smoking at around 20. (There are over 4000 chemicals in burning of a cigarette by the way, so I'd encourage anyone to quit). And so for years I'd been on low calorie or low fat diets. I did try keeping natural and 'healthy' (as I thought I could anyway), but the battle continued, and constantly gaining back more than what I'd lose would continue too. There were times, even when staying on diet I'd feel like I only had to *look* at food and I could gain weight! my *metabolism* getting slower . . . and slower . . . as the years went. I was told I had "borderline hypothyroidism", by one doctor, who also wanted to start me on a "little" medication that I'd have to have the rest of my life. I didn't like having to be on medication then either so I turned it down. Having "hypothyroidism" was also considered an "excuse" for one's weight problem at the time (as I actually was informed just recently as well)!

Then the low carb diet came along . . . Great! I can eat chicken with the skin! . . . and burghers! but, without the bun and mash potatoes! :p...::sigh::.. ok So I cut down on simple carbs, white sugar, white bread (which was a good thing) but the bad thing was *artificial* sweeteners in *diet* sodas and iced teas. However, constant hunger and cravings was always a problem I'd fall back on. Even if I were full I might still be thinking about food and what to have next. All along feeling 'guilty' :/ which made me feel 'bad' :(which I then 'remedied' by eating something good! :)

I did try 'ephedra' when it was out, being that it was 'natural' and actually that was the one thing that helped! I only had one in the morning and felt energized and good most of the day not thinking of food all day! Then, *that* of course, was soon taken off the market! hmmm I finally gave up on "dieting". The thought of *any* diet was just too much at that point. I knew I wouldn't be able to stay on anything for long, and I'd more than likely simply gain anything I lost (and more) right back! in fact I *knew* I would. I was just . . . plain . . . tired.

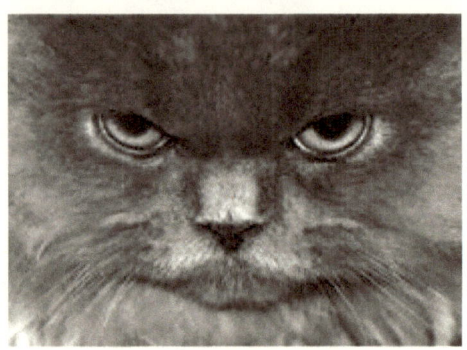

"Ok, enough of this . . ." . . . (I decided walking home from the train station after work one day). I totally had it with guilt, trying, failing, worrying about what anyone *else* said I should or shouldn't eat, how much I should or shouldn't have, how long I should or shouldn't exercise, should or shouldn't weigh etc. etc. etc. I just wanted to be *normal* about food and diet. I decided I'd still try to stay pretty much natural and as *"healthy"* as I thought I could anyway with whole foods, cooking from scratch and bringing my own lunches to work now (saving some money too), but I always did want to *go organic*. I used to get "Mother Earth News" and I actually did grow my own little organic garden for a few years. I even had *corn*! (Ok they were 5 inches long . . . but they were *my* corn! :) Unfortunately, I got away from it after having my two little ones to run around after, and then as a single mom, working full-time and just didn't have time for much of anything else actually.

Still living and working in New York in early 2007 I saw an organic grocery site that did home delivery in my area. I thought to myself "at least it may be a little more healthier for us". But, the draw also was that I could order right on line and it would cut shopping time! so this worked out great too. I'd even order or make organic desserts and snacks from scratch. *Nothing* was *"off the table"* so to speak:). *My diet, my way!* Just a regular menu without any counts, fats, weights or switches (after so many years of being on and off diets, this was a novelty to me). I now eat organic mostly whole grains such as brown rice, breads, and pasta. I buy organic dairy products (this is very important) and organic fruits and vegetables as much as I can, and every other month or so order free range grass fed meats and poultry. I now use *healthy* oils (very important), such as organic extra virgin olive oil, and just lately, organic coconut oil (my new healthy oil favorite!). Melted for oil, solid for a shortening or butter substitute sometimes when baking.

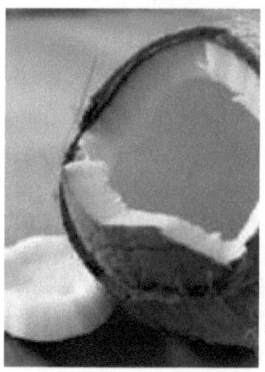

I did read how a doctor in the UK gave coconut oil to her husband who then showed remarkable improvement within weeks for *Alzheimers!* so it seems (in my opinion of course), to be something very good to include in my own diet as well! Your brain is 60% fat by the way, and the good fat in your brain helps create the cell membranes for the rest of the body. So getting *healthy* fats (such as coconut oil and olive oil) is vital. Omega 3s are also important here, (in grass fed beef, flax oil, cold water fish) for brain health, and, actually it may now be considered a deficiency and need in other mental disorders.

Just a few benefits reported of Coconut Oil

Infection fighter (a natural antibiotic)
Hair & Skin health
Weight Loss
Hypothyroidism
Bone Health
Alzheimer's Disease

*   *   *

Please Note: I would like to point out at this time, that vitamin *supplements* may indeed have allergy affects (in rare instances). Some vitamin supplements may also conflict with any medications you may be taking as well. Always consult with your doctor or health professional before taking them.

*   *   *

So What *Does* Organic Mean?

Organic produce and herbs are grown without the use of pesticides, synthetic fertilizers, sewage sludge, genetically modified organisms, or ionizing radiation. Animals that produce meat, poultry, eggs, and dairy products do not take antibiotics (or are used minamilly as I better understand) or growth hormones. Cows are grass fed, and chickens are free range. Organic eggs are darker in color as they have chickens exposed to more sunlight, and therefore more natural Vitamin D. You can check out the National Pesticide Information Center online for more information on what pesticides are allowed also. Another site would be whatsonmyfood.com to compare organic to non-organic produce.

The "Rustic" Glossary

Since I am not a medical, science or chemistry student (I'm sure you're surprised to hear:) for the sake of clarification and understanding, the following are my own definitions of a few important terms:

Chemicals and/or Toxins: Anything void of natural nutritive value and harmful to the body or environment, whether it be in, on, or around food or household products. This has been argued many times (*ad nauseum:*) and so I believe it needs to be defined as I see it here. I do not consider whole foods and nutrients to be *"chemicals"* or *"toxins"*. And I don't consider other 'safe' organic substances (such as baking soda) as *"toxins"* or *"chemicals"*. In the "Rustic Glossary", a *chemical* or *toxin* would be considered a synthetic chemical or *poison*, with more *harmful* effect on living things, as I believe it in the "risk/benefit" ratio.

Low immunity response: The body is reacting in a *weak* defensive way because it is not getting *enough* nutritive "reinforcements" to fight off disease. Allergies and disease (such as flus, colds and other viruses, asthma and other childhood diseases) are *a low* immunity response to outside intrusions (being carcinogenic, chemical and/or toxic, bacterial or viral), whether the "intrusions" be in foods, air, water, etc. and an indication of more healthy nutrients needed. (Vitamin C may be a big one here:).

Vitamin Supplements: Since *good* science and technology have made them available to us all (very appreciatively), vitamins and other nutrients can be found in "supplement" tablet form, with the understanding vitamins found in foods and as close to their natural whole composition work best with our body's natural living system. I do not consider (for the sake of the reader and this book) that vitamins in supplement form are "chemicals" or "toxins" *necessarily*. It would depend on their source. Some may very well be derived from unnatural synthetic sources (which I would consider *chemical or toxic* as defined above) so it is good to read labels and research what supplements are whole food sources and what supplements are not. (For instance D3 would be the natural source in supplement form, D2 would be the synthetic composition of vitamin D. The sun would be the best source! imo :)

Diet or Dieting: Pertaining to any study and finding of "dietary" health needs and effects and/or "weightloss" based on non-organic conventional foods and dieting for the most part today. Therefore, may or may not be or have the same effect as an "organic" diet or organic foods (in my opinion that is). For instance: regular coffee (how it is grown) may have more of an adverse effect on health than *organically* grown coffee (without chemical toxins). Some do say I am *"in denial"* on this however:)

_____

_____

Chapter 2

It's Not Just About Me

Allergies, Arthritis and Asthma Buzz Off!

The person who says it cannot be done should not interrupt the person doing it.

Chinese Proverb.

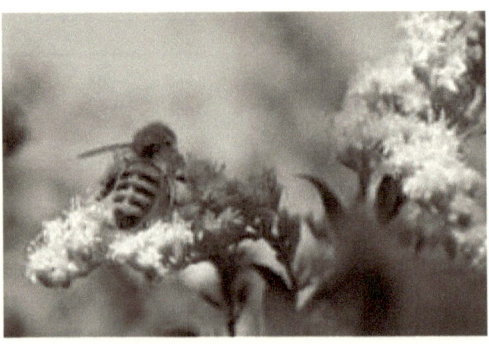

These three, allergies, arthritis and asthma, seem to be the easiest (in my opinion anyway) to say "Buzz off" to now, in a very effective way naturally, with whole nutrients and an *organic* diet! (Just going by my own experience and reading quite a bit of others). Actually, diabetes and high blood pressure are right behind them! and it really saddens and amazes me at the same time to see the still prevalence of them today and how many more "new and improved" drugs come out to deal with them. It does feel like a different world when I see commercials about them now (please pay close attention to the list of side-effects in them).

Now again, I am not speaking as a medical professional but what allergies and asthma mean to me is *a low* immune system reaction, and *too many toxins* (as defined in the "Rustic Glossary"). It is a little confusing, as I understand in conventional teaching it is the opposite actually, being an elevated immune system response. And, what arthritis means to me is a lack of nutrients and too many (inflammatory?) *toxins*. I completely understand there are varying stages and degrees of symptoms, so some might take a little longer than others to remedy, but nutrients and *eliminating* the underlying *cause* of them all (to begin with) is getting on the right track. Basically, it is a rethinking of health, diet and remedies than you've probably been told.

I was also diagnosed with arthritis in my lower back several years ago. That's when I began taking calcium supplements (with magnesium and Vit. D) everyday, and have not needed any thing else for arthritis since! However, keep in mind this was at the very *beginning* of my problem with it, so it may take a little more time and other nutrients to help if you have a worse case, but! you *can* get relief and help naturally! without added medications and pain killers. My doctor would ask me every once in a while how my back was doing, and I would say "o . . . it's ok" . . . not going into my "experiments" anymore with nutrients, as well she thought it was amusing when I did try to tell her, but at least she didn't scowl "You get enough vitamins in your food!" so I liked her. Her and Dr. Lee, before he retired. I'd ask him if I could try something or other, an herb I remember one time for weight loss. He laughed and said, "Sure! . . . it won't work . . . but sure!" . . . Well, he was right about that one anyway :)

So, how did I know to take calcium supplements anyway? Some years earlier, the mother-in-law of a friend was having a lot of pain with arthritis in her arms (and you could see the difficulty she was having on her face). At the time I had only *heard* calcium supplements were good for arthritis (probably from my mom). My mom used to read "Prevention" magazine, and took vitamins every day herself . . . (her eyesight actually got *better* as she got older and had to take her glasses *off* to read, so I'm guessing from the vitamins she took too). I simply told her what I had heard about calcium. She actually went out and took my advice! (I wasn't used to someone taking *my* advice then or now actually:) She went out and got calcium supplements, and told me *happily* how . . . "they worked!" and how she felt so much better! when I saw her again a few months later. I was so happy for her (and just as surprised actually, not really knowing for myself at the time) simply hoping it might help. I hate seeing people in pain (I can't take much of it myself).

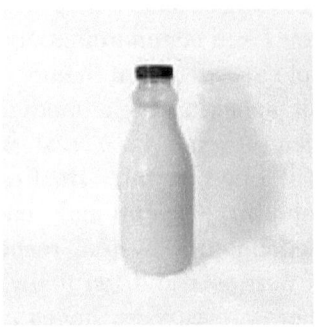

One grandmother is worth two M.D.s :)

I do wish conventional doctors would not dismiss natural alternative remedies so easily! (If they do that is). Proper diagnosing is great, but remedying with more body-friendly *"first, do no harm"* nutrients, herbs, vitamins seem to me to be much better. "Calcium deficiency and low bone mineral density is found to be common in patients with rheumatoid arthritis." One study (alternative I suppose:) looked at the use of calcium and vitamin D supplements in patients with juvenile rheumatoid arthritis and found that calcium supplementation along with vitamin D significantly increased the bone mineral density in these patients. I think that's awesome! The notable thing is, I found out about the studies *after the fact* . . . after experiencing personally calcium worked for arthritis.

Some other benefits of Calcium?

Calcium strengthens bones, protects cardiac muscles, prevents colon cancer, prevents premenstrual blues, prevents kidney stones, ensures healthy alkaline pH level, controls blood pressure (nice!), maintains healthy teeth and gums, and helps transportation of nutrients. So, it's yet another "multi tasker"!

It is also important to take a calcium supplement *with* magnesium, as magnesium will help your body absorb calcium correctly. I have a calcium supplement with both magnesium and Vitamin D right now. My son actually grinds up his own (organic) egg shells to a powder for a natural source of calcium also.

A little about Magnesium

I'm just hearing a little about magnesium and how it may be another "super-nutrient" that is critically needed in *almost every tissue and system* in the entire body! Deficiencies in it have caused muscle weakness and atrophy, brittle bones (good for the elderly?) unnecessarily high heart rates, poor blood sugar metabolism, and a host of other problems. Magnesium deficiencies can lead to poor arterial health, which directly causes high blood pressure. So it is important to be sure you're getting enough magnesium as well with your calcium.

~~~~~~

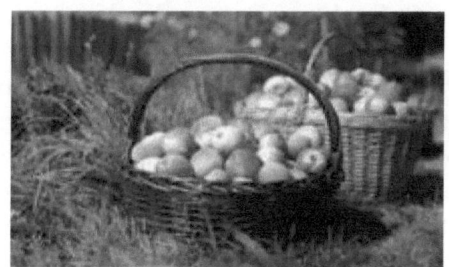

Calcium (with magnesium to absorb) is just one way to help with arthritis. Apple cider vinegar is also one that has great results. A woman in her 50's in a news article from the UK with *crippling* arthritis, (unable to even go to the store and shopping at the time), was told by her daughter to look into apple cider vinegar and honey (natural anti-inflammatories?). She did try it for herself, and was up and fine after nothing else was working for her! I think that's pretty awesome (I wonder now if having more organic apples will help prevent arthritis). *"An apple a day"* . . . hmmmm

Some other benefits of apple cider vinegar? just to name a few are: it kills head lice (instead of those chemical filled shampoos I hesitantly used on my poor sons once thinking that was the *only way)* it reverses aging! yes! It eases digestion, and washes "toxins" from the body (very important). Helps also with obesity and diabetes. I use it as a cold remedy along with honey and cinnamon very effectively as well. You can think of it for your pets also, to help get rid of fleas *without* harmful chemicals perhaps. And, it also helped someone I spoke with online regarding their . . . hemorrhoids (!) . . .

"wow . . . thankyou! crystbear! (crystbear is my old "retired" nic, 2 days later) **as soon as you said yeast infection, i knew it . . . that's what it felt like originally coming on, but i knew they were hemorroids and i didn't put the two together. i immediately applied acv directly and while it burned it was nothing compared to the burning insatible itch . . . i'm so happy i think i can handle this w/o a doctor. :)"physician heal thyself". i've also started to drink acv..**

it's something i've wanted to have in my diet anyway..also just going forward with as raw and fresh as possible . . . peace"

Well wow! I was so happy for her and so happy that she came back to tell me too. Once again I had no idea whether something would actually work (or one would actually take my advice) in this case apple cider vinegar for hemorrhoids, but . . . there it is! I also now wonder if nutrients can help with substance abuse problems as well? Not *saying* it positively, just wondering?

Amazing Apple Cider Vinegar has also been used for:

Acid reflux, acne, allergies (including pollen, food, pet and environmental), arthritis, asthma, hypertension (high blood pressure) candida, cholesterol problems, chronic fatigue, dermatitis, eczema, fungal infections like athlete's foot, jock itch and nail fungus, gout, influenza, sinus infection, and sore throat! One in "Testimonials" you will see did use it on her eczema, and how it worked after many years of trying everything else. Eh, just a few little things :)

Use organic raw unpasteurised ACV (apple cider vinegar) with the cloudy "mother". When it is raw (unpasteurised) it contains valuable enzymes, and when you use ACV always dilute with water or juice when drinking it.

I would absolutely keep a bottle of organic raw apple cider vinegar in the house! (and I don't believe you have to consult anyone on that:)

Bee Pollen, Allergies and Cholesterol

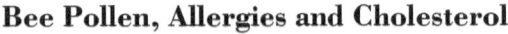

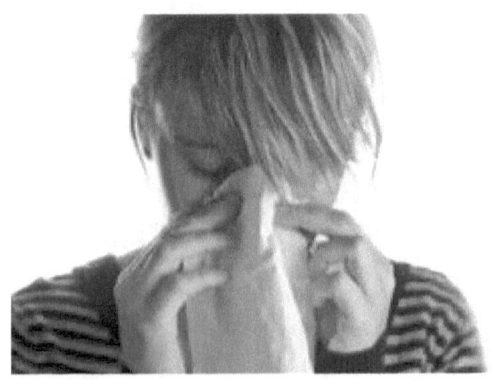

My youngest son had a *lot* of trouble with asthma as a child (in the hospital many times for it) then allergies for years has now since taking vitamins, organic bee pollen granules, (an amazing multi-nutrient source)

and changing his diet also to wholefood organic, totally stopped all sneezing, sinus congestion (and we're in the middle of the country with constant high pollen count). He believed it was also from dust or something in the vents when the heat came on, and I used to wonder why I wasn't as affected as he was, but I was also taking vitamins (especially a lot of C) for some years and for years he dismissed anything I said about them. I actually did the same when my mom would read about them so I understand. I mean I *heard* her when she would read out loud something or other, but I didn't take them for myself . . . until I was finally on 4 meds for my asthma! So I guess that's how it goes :) Now he's more serious than I am on healthy organic food and nutrients! Raw bee pollen was one that he read about himself and began taking it at about the same time taking vitamins and going organic. Bee pollen may desensitize some individuals against airborne pollen by consuming trace amounts over a period of weeks or months. It may be more effective if the beehive exists within a few miles of your home, though my son purchased organic raw bee pollen online. Bee pollen also contains all the nutrients needed to survive alone on (interestingly if you had enough of it I suppose). So, I wonder if that also doesn't help people with their allergies? by strengthening the immune system with all the nutrients needed as well.

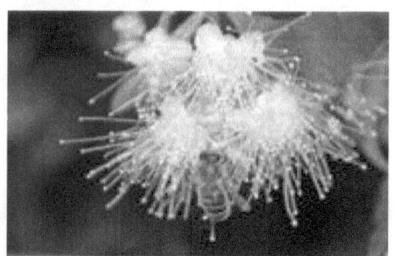

A few other benefits of Bee Pollen

I came across this testimony regarding one's cholesterol level and bee pollen granules:

. . . . "my cholestrol results were 246. I was scheduled to return in two weeks for retesting. During those two weeks, I took . . . fresh bee pollen granules (each) day. My cholestrol test results returned at 146. I don't think any prescription meds can do that. My doctor was dumbfounded and asked what I had done different. She documented that I had taken bee pollen and had tremendous results."

Bee pollen has *multi* benefits to be looked into as well not only for allergies, but perhaps for cholesterol too. Since high cholesterol is so prevalent today I thought I'd share that. Bee pollen granules are also high in vitamins, minerals and protein. They support red-blood-cell efficiency and are a possible anti-aging supplement. Athletes use it for energy support. I do take it every once in a while as a multi-vitamin source personally.

It should be noted that some may indeed have very bad allergic reaction to bee pollen as well, so be sure to consult with your doctor first. I took just a few granules to be sure I had no reaction.

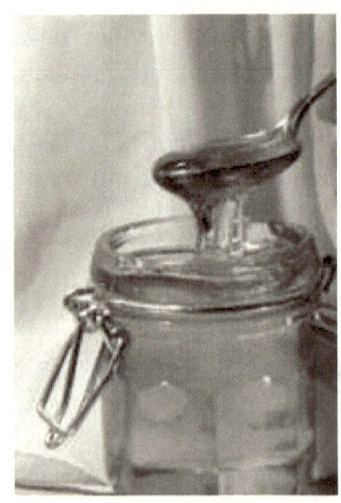

Just a little about Honey (another super-food?!) . . .

Along with bee pollen, there are many health benefits of organic raw *honey*. Honey can be a powerful immune system booster as well. I take it the first slightest sign of a soar throat and cold. It's antioxidant and anti-bacterial properties can also help improve digestive system and help you stay healthy and fight disease. A suggestion for a natural cleansing tonic is: Mix a spoonful of honey and lemon juice from half a lemon into a cup of warm water and drink it before breakfast.

I would look into getting *organic raw* especially, as non-organic honey has a high concentrated amount of pesticides in it which unfortunately is the reason for "colony collapse". When I first heard how bees were 'disappearing' mysteriously, it took a few minutes to think "hmmm pesticides?", then several years later it was found yep . . . *pesticides* :/ Yet *another* sad effect of toxins and chemicals in the environment, and yet another reason to go organic would be to help save our own *natural* ecological system from being *totally* ruined by *unnatural* and *unnecessary* chemicals and pesticides contributing to it (by the billions of pounds every year). So, it goes hand in hand. Cleaning our environment, and eliminating toxins from going into us as well. (Simply going organic would be a great way to help as well in my opinion).

"If we doctors threw all our medicines into the sea, it would be that much better for our patients and that much worse for the fishes." Oliver Wendell Holmes, M.D.

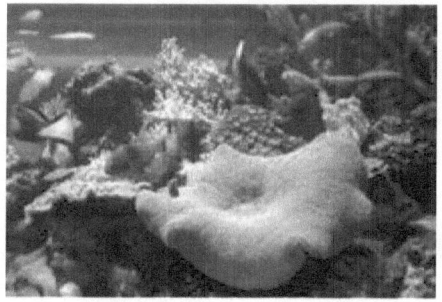

Chapter 3

Go Organic Or . . .

How to get healthy, be happy (*and* lose weight?) without really trying :)

Disease is the censor pointing out the humans, animals and plants who are imperfectly nourished. Wrench, G. T. The Wheel of Health, 1941. London: Daniel, p 130.

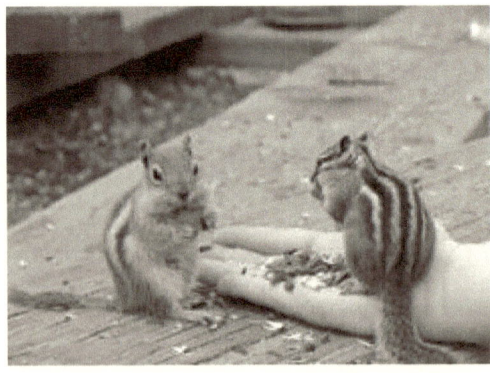

It seems (to me anyway) most all of nature knows what to do about food and dieting! Have you ever thought about that? How do animals know what to eat, when to eat, how much to eat, and when to stop? It is absolutely amazing to me, and interesting, that everything in nature knows how to do these things . . . *except us apparently!* Hmmmm We have all kinds of "dietary" plans, disciplines, taboos, cravings, addictions and more (if I hear one more . . . :/). And that seems (to me) only in the last 50 or so years, especially in America. I used to look at some nice skinny people sitting down simply picking and choosing what they wanted, and I was so envious. Or, my sons could gobble down five times more and not gain an ounce! I *could look* at food and it would instantly cause weight gain! (only those with a weight problem can relate to this I'm afraid). I know one may say, "It's your *metabolism*!". Ok, but what makes *my* "*metabolism*" different from another's "*metabolism*"? Well this is the one thing that I stumbled upon that helped me begin to at least lose weight, that I could not do all these years . . . I went *Organic*. You might have guessed it by now (you probably did actually:) but I'm going to show you how, and hopefully convince you here and throughout the rest of this book why you should (including natural cosmetics and household cleaning products) go organic! as much as possible, whether you have a weight problem or not!

Fact is, I do believe the cause of a *lot* of weight and health problems in America is *not* too many calories, carbs and fats *necessarily*, but *too many toxins*, and *how organic* food (with *less* toxins) does *actually metabolize* better. Or that illnesses and ailments do not just *mysteriously* come upon us or "jump in us". These are the seven that seem to be the most prevalent (nowadays anyway): 1. Allergies 2. Asthma 3. Arthritis 4. Diabetes 5. Heart disease 6. High blood pressure and 7. *Cancer*. I guess you can add Obesity to that, although new and unheard of ailments are now seemingly turning up every day, and just as *mysteriously* ("Morgellons? being one of them . . . please look that one up, it's *scary*). Going into health & healing forums wanting to share what I've learned (or think I've learned:) for the last year is where I hear about many of them. The causes I believe are *unnatural* things used in our own supposedly "healthy" regular food supply and/ or environment. (clue: gmos, free radicals, *toxins*) to begin with, wearing down our immune system, and the effects come out in various ways. Do you ever wonder how medicine has grown so "advanced" and yet so *incapable* of getting rid of disease? Hormones and antibiotics (in poultry and cattle) preservatives and chemical pesticides (*Poisons* . . . they *Kill*) and chemical fertilizers (i.e. *toxins*, billions of pounds each year, that's *billions* with a "*b*") producing foods (and environments) that are not in their natural (organic) good-for-us state. This is interesting. It is now warned how grapefruit juice can "interfere" with medications, and people are told to not have it if they're on medication (not sure if that is for certain meds or all meds). But, I heard the doctor say this, that the body "prefers the grapefruit juice", (that caught my attention) and so that's what it takes first, *rejecting* the medication. I thought that was so interesting . . . so the body itself knows what's good for it!

How do non-organic produced foods cause you to gain weight? (or keep you from losing weight?) Well, hormones and antibiotics are given to animals to *increase* their appetite and gain weight *faster*. So now, *what* would that be doing to many of us when we ingest them? All this recent talk and concern about *"Obesity in America"! "Obesity in America"!* Some medications (made from or contain toxins) themselves may be the cause of weight gain and other ailments and illnesses as well.

I have found in this last year, that this is indeed *not* readily received well by *everyone!* When I went into dieter's forums trying to share what I found (or believed I found) was good news, it was quickly put down and dashed, :("Misinformation!" "Heretic!" . . . When I wrote about it to some well known "diet gurus" and a few others, I never did get a response :(I actually thought it would be *Great News?!* But, no I found out otherwise! Just the contrary actually :/ So, it's not for those who do like, and can live on regular (i.e. low cal, low fat, low carb, counts, weights, eat less/exercise more, BMI charts, etc.) diets, and even have 'conquered' their battle with diet and exercise on their own! Cool! Or with hours and $$ spent on weekly support groups, perhaps years in therapy over *guilt* and your 'inability to control' 'undisciplined' obsessive compulsive . . . blah blah :) Or you hire your own personal trainer like Osmin! (my son loves that show) He *is* inspiring, but I tried for years, and could not maintain it for long each time on my own. I would *still encourage* you to *go organic* to get and keep *toxins* out of your system (as much as one can anyway) for your *health's sake*! (which will be explained too). However, I know there are many many more out there (actually millions more) who don't understand what they are going through. The constant battle, the constant guilt, of constantly *trying to diet*, metabolism getting slower, exercise, yet having the incessant draw back to overeating and bingeing (like the chickens and cows). Or perhaps just losing your will to even try anymore (as I did). Either that or even more fun?! *Not* overeating and bingeing but, actually eating less, exercising more, and still not losing! Perhaps another side-effect of non-organic toxins in foods that can affect you that way as well? Probably asking yourself "Is this all there is?" "Will it ever be 'normal'?" atleast as far as 'weight control and diet' is concerned? Yes! Here's the *happy* news you have been waiting for. Organic foods are more *efficiently* digested by your body (like the grapefruit juice?) because you *don't have* the toxins to process also (or as many anyway). Your body will process food better, you'll not have a major problem of overeating or craving, (like the CAFOs) and you will have a sense of normalcy and control again with the ability to pick and choose (like the skinny people I envied so much) without guilt or stress or feeling of deprivation either (just like all of nature too?).

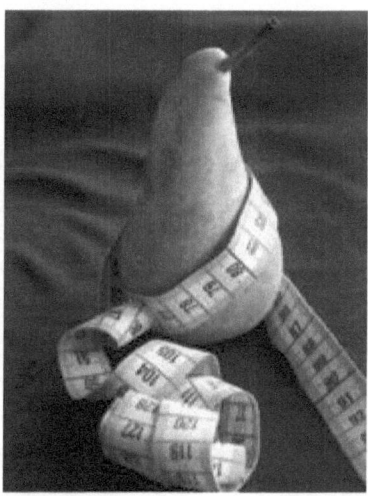

So many I've spoken to in diet forums are totally convinced it must be an eat less/exercise more diet and fitness program, and that's fine! If you're worried about 'Dieting gone wild'? to that I would say simply "F*ollow whatever diet you wish*'! only make it with *organic* (without the added *toxins*) food and maybe see for yourself if it helps (at least to stay on your diet). My main focus now however, is *not* on losing weight *alone*, but how to *get healthy* (I know that get's people ripping mad! ;) The thing is I have lost some weight thus far (35+ lbs) not 'dieting' per se, but *only* by changing my food to healthy organic foods, and the miracle being I have not gained it back. Um, yes, even chocolate and real desserts (hey, they could be healthy!:) It's easy to make your own from any recipe (*just use organic ingredients!*). I've had thus far no restrictions other than it being *organic* healthy and (try to be) balanced. Real food, (protein, vegetable, fruit) just regular menus, but what's happened is, (and this is important) I no longer crave! or have hunger pangs all day, as I did most of my adult life to battle! Very *naturally*, I could eat less, and could actually stop at one piece of organic berry pie, or organic chocolate cake easily because I no longer have the incessant desire to eat half the cake every time no matter how full I am :/ :)

If . . . there . . . is . . . anything . . . I'd like to do here it's to free someone from a real obsession with simply *trying* to lose weight alone. I believe the stress and guilt along with it may *work against* you also. (For pity's sake, who doesn't want to be thin??) Get off of "dieting" (I really don't even like the topic for weight loss anymore:p) and on to eating *"healthy organic"* for *your health's* sake! The help here is, you will no longer have too many hormones and antibiotics in your system working *against* you either affecting your *metabolism.* "Excessive estrogen (sprayed on non-organic produce and given to poultry and cattle) causes the body to *become more* insulin-resistant (diabetic too? hmmm) and creates *more fat cells*", great! and by eliminating it will help you stay *on any diet you like!* if you like! Not only will you live longer and be healthier, you'll live *happier!* I have read there is evidence that indicates organic food is also more nutritious (though this has been refuted but sorry not to my satisfaction anyway). I do not believe *toxins* could have absolutely no effect on nutritive value personally, and the lack of hazardous toxins helps your body perform more efficiently as nature intended. "You then are able to convert the organic food into the full energy potential. This translates to less fatigue and having the extra energy needed to burn off even more calories." Well that's good news isn't it?!

It also apparently means less heartburn too! Since I used to get it two or three times a week at least on regular foods, my stomach protesting the toxins (I didn't know it at the time) it was given to process. That's what *"indigestion" is!* (so I found out for myself) *too many toxins* and your body creating too *much acid to digest them* (where ulcers come from? where "inflammation" comes from?) hmmm At the time I'd take a calcium supplement for it (which worked by the way). When I heard in the commercial how 'Tums' had *calcium* in it, I thought to myself . . . "I wonder if calcium alone will help?" and . . . it did!) however, now I have not had to take any, because organic food metabolizes better (because of less toxins and therefore less acid indigestion!). There's another benefit of going organic!

So yes you *can* have real organic (without hormones, antibiotics, pesticides) cheese and dairy (perhaps). I know, at least it seems, more and more people are "lactose intolerant" these days, but now I personally wonder if that's what some may *be intolerant of*? to begin with. Not sure, just wondering? I'm thinking it fits in my own "hypothesis" that allergies may be a nutrient deficiency or an over toxic condition and environment in general. And so yes, I believe we *can* rethink all kinds of 'dietary needs', ailments and taboos set upon us all by conventional medicine, food, and diet gurus alike :) . . . like . . . this . . .

"Healthy" Organic Dark Chocolate Cake *Recipe!

INGREDIENTS

For the chocolate cake:

1/2 cup organic cocoa (I found online)
hot water and organic milk
1 cup unbleached organic flour
1/2 tsp sea salt
1 tsp baking soda

4 tbsp organic coconut oil
1 cup organic raw sugar
1 organic egg yoke
1 tsp organic vanilla extract

PREPARATION:

Preheat oven to 350 degrees. Butter and flour an 8 X 8 cake pan

In a 1 cup measure, put cocoa powder. Add enough hot water for the powder to dissolve mixed with a fork, and then fill the rest of the cup up with milk.

Combine flour, salt, and baking soda, mixing well with a fork.

Beat coconut oil and sugar, add egg yolk, beating for one minute. Stir in vanilla and combine everything.

Mix for one minute. Turn batter into buttered pan.

Bake for about 35 minutes or until cake tests done. Place on a cooling rack.

Dust with organic powdered sugar (yes it is available online) or for a quick and easy chocolate icing (if you wish) though the cake is rich and moist alone, I sometimes make a simple gnache (chopped organic dark chocolate, a little heavy cream, a little organic sugar and vanilla, and add 1 tablespoon of instant coffee melted together in sauce pan carefully or in a bowl over simmering water) pour on top of cake when cooled. Serve with unsweetened whipped cream (if you so wish). Now, I'm sure I'm going to hear a barrage of protests from conventional "diet gurus", but I might have this every once in a while. Why? because I no longer have the *cravings* I had on any and all the non-organic low-fat, low-carb, low-cal food *diets!* That's why! That's what makes *me* happy anyway?! I have what I choose to have, when I choose to have it! . . . And for some more *healthy happy news?* . . .

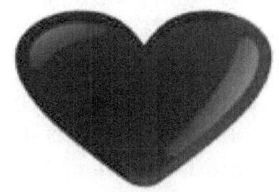

Chocolate Lowers Blood Pressure

Eating moderate amounts of dark chocolate can help reduce blood pressure (well that works for me!). It is found that individuals that consistently ate dark chocolate had lower risks of heart problems, including high blood pressure, when compared to those that avoided chocolate! hmmmm:) Scientists think that a compound found in high amounts in chocolate, known as flavonoids, relax vascular tissue, thus lowering blood pressure!

So, who says desserts can't be healthy?! :)

*There's a very *controversial* Dark Chocolate Banana Treat recipe (on Rustic's Healthy Recipes at the end of this book also:) I spoke of it once, had it once, and I heard about it for weeks and weeks afterward in forum online :/ I'm "*slathering in it*" now! :) . . . No *I don't* have it every day, I don't have it hardly ever! (no longer having craving off-the-wall problems) but, once in a while I will have a "rustic healthy" (*albeit* controversial:) treat! :))

But, what about the sugar?

I know some are thinking "But, what about the '*sugar*'?! *What about the sugar?! . . . Rustic?? . . . Heretic!!" (please see also my commentary "The New Scapegoat:)* Well this is very interesting, I found out that molasses (the part *removed* leaving regular white sugar?) is the part *that contains* the *healthy nutrients!* in it (including iron), and left in it's whole state the body processes *organic* sugar with less effect (less spike in insulin level I would say? don't know, don't have a lab of my own yet :) (and I'm not a scientist, biologist or chemist:) than white sugar alone because it is in it's whole form? (like whole grain bread rather than white bread perhaps?) What started me thinking about this was when I read someone actually taking molasses to help out with her iron level to gain energy, and it ended up curing her tinnitus as well! So I wondered "hmmmm, is sugar in it's *whole organic form* (with the molasses part) perhaps *not* one of the *culprits afterall??*" Whole source organic sugar is not bad (in my opinion) Ok Ok . . . "*In Moderation*" (before someone tips and falls back on their computer seat:) or wants to "reach in their computer and smack me" . . . (it gets rough in health forums sometimes:) but then when you go organic your cravings will stop! and *you will* then be able to eat "*In Moderation*" and not because someone else *tells you to*. That's what I believe is the great news here! You won't need anyone *telling* you what you can or can't have. Your *endocrine system* (the body's *hormonal* system . . . ha! see I *can* learn!:) will naturally regulate itself (and your *metabolism)* since it's getting what it needs *naturally*, and so now you can *"Get healthy, be happy, (and lose weight perhaps?) without really trying!"* :)

(Organic) Black Strap Molasses I have it, but rarely use it . . . may start now! Please note: I did read to take it with food or protein, the iron in it may be too strong for your stomach. Molasses is one of those amazing foods that has good health effects on many things by the way (not only for energy). It has been reported as a natural remedy for the following:

restless leg syndrome

chronic fatigue

arthritic pain and swelling   acne
joint pains

heart palpatations

increased bone density   nose

bleeds

source of potassium

circulation

nails are stronger

constipation

swelling in ankles and hands   blood sugar

levels

and apparently for someone's tinnitus too! wow

Organic vs. Conventional the difference

An interesting thing to note is the three countries that eat the most organic foods per capita are Denmark, Switzerland and Austria. According to the CIA World Factbook Denmark, Switzerland and Austria are all in the top 25 percent ranking of countries with the highest life expectancies.

"A person must have a certain amount of intelligent ignorance to get anywhere." Charles F. Kettering

Chapter 4

It Takes Time

This guy's doctor told him he had six months to live. The guy said he couldn't pay his bill. The doctor gave him another six months. :)

Henny Youngman

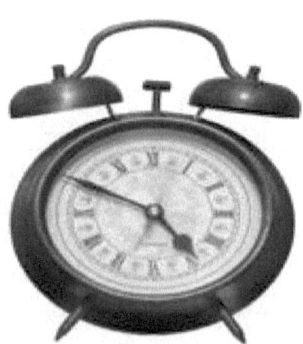

Getting healthy and/or losing weight may take a little time for you to notice results. *Of course* it would depend on your particular individual health condition, situation and food availability and choices. *Needless* to say I'm sure, eating a more healthy fresh fruit and vegetable diet will make you healthier or lose weight a little faster?! (as we're told *ad nauseum:*) Everyone in the world probably knows that by now I'm sure as well. *The problem* is having the consistent long-term actual will and *ability to do* so. (Try telling that to the myriad specialists and *diet gurus:*). I also know we would all want an *instant pill* and some may work! (like ephedra) natural or not, but only for the time you take them. You won't want to hear this but, you'll only find yourself right back where you started and unfortunately perhaps worse as you're still *not* getting the nutrients you really do need to begin with to help your body heal itself. Or the side effects of the one pill or substance has now caused *another* ill effect and now you have even more problems. Please consider carefully that your body *is not meant* for nutrient-void chemicals and heavy metals (all those ingredients you can't pronounce) other than those found in natural whole foods and nutrients. Am I against the food industry and free capitalism? Of course not! I'm only asking that they use wholesome healthy ingredients too in what they create and sell. I'd buy them! I am noticing more and more organic choices now though, so that is great news and I thank the companies big or small that are doing it!

So, whether you have a weight (or 'wait') problem it probably won't be instant coffee:) But I will say, you will be a lot better healthwise and happier going this way; no longer being *'obsessed'* or *guilt* ridden. So *relax!* Have a cup of *organic* coffee (sans the pesticides), with real organic (containing healthy molasses part) sugar and organic milk (sans the hormones and antibiotics) and a piece of that organic (now *good* for you:) *chocolate* cake . . . and enjoy! I noticed for myself it did take a few weeks before I began to no longer *crave* or have hunger all day, or sometimes even *think* of food many times. I tried it two different occasions, actually, on three . . .

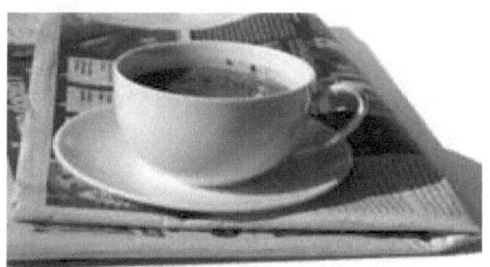

The first was when I water fasted for 8 days. I didn't put it together then that being the first "detox" experience. After fasting, I felt energized and no more cravings for food and increase of appetite (for a little while anyway). I did not realize it was the 'natural' (what I thought "healthy") fruit and vegetables, dairy and meats (low fat, low cal, low carb or not) non-organic food *itself* that had the toxins to detox *from*, and actually helped *cause* the cravings and increase appetite to begin with, and to slowly return once again. And so when I went back to regular food and diet the guilt and battle continued! After going organic for several months I kept thinking "Boy, this is weird?!" not actually looking for or thinking of food all day! (the same as I felt after water fasting). I lost about 15 lbs. then (keeping in mind all the years I *tried* to lose weight, yet I only *gained* weight right back and more). However at that time I didn't pay attention to the length of time it took before the cravings stopped (because I never expected it could happen!).

We then moved down to Virginia, and I returned to buying regular "healthy" food not having home delivery, and once again, my usual cravings returned. Deciding to return once again for the second time to organic, I paid closer attention and took note this time. The first few weeks it was the same and so I thought, "Well, maybe I'm wrong" a little disappointed. Maybe it *was* a "*placebo* effect" afterall, back to constantly feeling hungry again, always thinking of what to have next. But after those first few weeks it did happen again! once again no longer feeling hungry and craving all day. So I am supposing it took that time to get the hormones and antibiotics out of my own system.

What brought it to my attention initally? What was it precisely *in* the non-organic "healthy" foods that caused the problem? (I wondered to myself also). Well, when I relayed what happened to the landlord at the ranch where we had moved, I was told how in conventional food production the chickens and cattle (I now know as CAFOs: Concentrated Animal Feeding Operations) were regularly injected with hormones and antibiotics for the very purpose to *eat more, gain weight and to get fatter faster*! "Oh?! hmmm" . . . I had not heard that before.

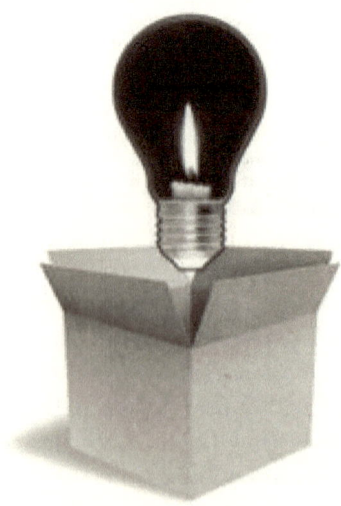

And so that's how the light went on :) and I began to put 2 + 2 together as to what the problem was all these years. Could it be that the same effect that occurred in the CAFO poultry and cows happened to me also? It was still kind of hard to believe at first. The thing is it doesn't affect *everyone* the same apparently (which is part of the deception I suppose). They don't affect everyone *the same*, but they *do* affect *everyone*! If not in weight gain and increased appetite, then in some other way (my son's headaches and allergies for instance) considering all the various diseases upon us (but more on that in "What do we Get"). And so I got on the internet searching to see if there were any other information I could find on it, and did come across a few articles giving actual details as to what happens as well. I then went into diet forums armed with some of the information, and to share some of what I had found! (thinking this was great news?!). After a few long "discussions" with some highly indignant diet forum 'leaders' with their "eat less/exercise more, that's it!" belief, rejecting what I was trying to share whenever I'd try to help some others who came in looking for help (having the same hard time staying on a diet as I did) however, in the middle of one lengthy "discussion":) another did tell me how she was helped by going organic also! . . .

"Thanks Crystbear! Yes, I've experienced weight loss just by switching to organic meats and dairy. The growth hormones fed to chickens, cattle, pigs . . . are a huge problem for our bodies . . . . adding tenacious fat-clinging calories. I feel sorry for all the children who balloon out just from eating normally and drinking milk loaded with these hormones."

Needless to say I was so very happy about that, and to actually hear from someone else personally who experienced the same as I did! and was trying to share.

Regarding added vitamins and nutrients, what I usually hear is "O, you get enough vitamins in your food" which is always curious to me to say not being possible to know what anyone else's diet is like everyday? or what one may need more than the other? How does anyone know that for someone else? My personal belief now is, unless you live in a perfect tropical climate picking your own (organic) nutrient rich foods everyday (FDA says 9 servings now, it used to be 5 I think) most might probably need additional vitamins and nutrients (from other whole food sources). But that is my opinion only. My thinking is if you're getting sick, you may not be getting enough of or the right nutrients afterall? I still take Vit. C, D, and Calcium supplements and some others daily. And, it may very well take a little time. It took a month or so for my son to see the difference in his allergies. I actually haven't had a real cold in over 4 years (except for the following

1 hour cold incident, which I will demonstrate how I handle them now :) and I've always been *very susceptible* to them, at least two or three a year if not more. So, you may see an improvement in that too, or guess what? You may just find yourself not being a *craving hungry lunatic anymore!* (like the CAFO chickens and cows:) . . .

~~~~~~

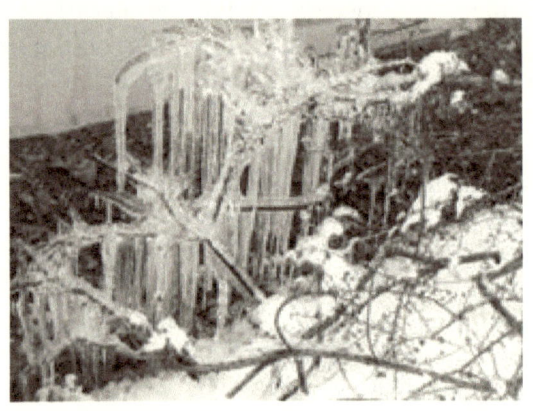

The 1 Hour Cold Melee

This sneak attack came on quick . . . *and strong.* It had been over 3 years since my last cold and asthma "attack" so it was rather unexpected. It was a cold winter (Jan. 2012) here in Virginia, and we keep thermostat on 58 (55 @ night trying to keep the cost down) and I'm susceptible in the cold. (I believed that's why they call it "cold and flu season" though I've been told I'm mistaken. Please see my commentary "On the Cold War Front" also:). While sitting at the computer on a usual uneventful day, it came on without warning. All kinds of 'bombardments' seemingly all at once too. First sneezing, then coughing, a little sore throaty, wheezing, headachey, chills, my head felt heavier and heavier by the minute. I honestly had never experienced it quite like that before all at the same time (I usually get a little warning such as a slight sore throat or something). "Oh, boy", remembering the days of colds, flu, and bronchial asthma attacks. Is it a cold? is it the flu? I do not know, but, I determined since I had already taken my regular "troop" of vitamins and nutrients, for this one (whichever it was, cold or flu, I still do not know, but it was something respiratory) I had to send in . . . yes . . . *Reinforcements!* and it had to be quick! As my head was now literally down to the keyboard I pushed my way from the desk and began to muster defense in this way, with what I had *ready, willing, able and waiting close at hand* (in the fridge and cupboard) . . .

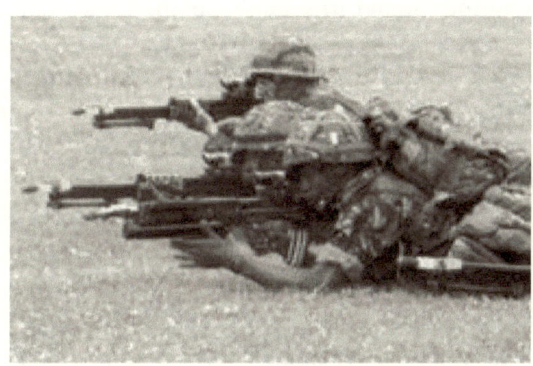

1 tsp. (organic) apple cider vinegar (natural anti-viral, antiseptic, alkalizing) sinuses and breathing felt a little better followed by: 1 tsp. (raw organic) honey (natural anti-bacterial healing) and throat felt a little better with (organic) ceylon cinnamon 1/4 tsp. or so sprinkled on top of the honey (a powerful natural antibiotic)

Did that round of three a few times . . . then sent in one of the *Big Guns*: yes . . . Vitamin C 1000! (with it's partners Bioflavanoids and Rosehips:) my stealth fav, that always comes through for me! *A natural antihistamine and immunity builder.* And, I made a cup of nice hot organic black tea (to help me warm up).

With the situation seeming to "stabilize", the nutrients doing their good work, yet still feeling somewhat drained, I then retreated to let the "reinforcements" finish the job, and laid down to watch some t.v. instead. Nothing takes me away from the computer much, but this strong "sneak attack" did . . . for about an hour that is (that's actually longer than my usual engagements) so this was the "1 Hour Cold Melee" and . . . *Battle Over!* I got up, and went back to my computer "station" . . . *"I . . . Feel . . . Better!" :))*

~~~~~~

Ok, sorry if that was a little short . . . *but . . . that was it!* If it had to take longer, I would have "reloaded", "repeat", and add some flaxseed oil (to help fight any infection) and another C1000 perhaps. I then tried sharing that when I was back online (yes mistakenly albeit:) and actually spent a *grueling half hour* (almost worse than the "1 Hour Cold Melee" itself) trying to tell one poster whom doubts everything I say, that I *did know* what a cold was! and *when* I was coming down with one! It's kind of fun on the health forums sometimes! What's strange to me is how some are so *sure* they just *know* that something can't be so! Even though they've never tried it or seen it for *themselves.* I mean I don't *believe everything* I read or hear? but if someone gives *their own* (even according to them) "anecdotal" experience, I'd still say "hmmm well, I'll see" or . . . "hmmm . . . I really don't know about that, maybe I'll look into it?!" . . . or something like that? So it was kind of strange and unexpected to me in the beginning sharing some of these things and the responses (battles, threats and attacks over them literally:) I've gotten :/ It's now been over a year since the "1 Hour Cold Melee", and I still have not had a cold, flu, or asthma problem since (thankfully). Now I am fully aware I can get sick at *any* time, if I am not ready! One thing I found about colds and flu is you do have to catch them as early as possible, since it seems to me it is more difficult to turn around once it takes hold. Please also bear in mind, I'm taking vitamins every day. Also, I am mostly organic now (so less "free radicals" for my body to fight off as well). Personally, I believe everything works together to help get and stay healthy, and why perhaps just one extra Vit. C1000 along with the other healthy natural food nutrients worked so well that time. As in the military men are prepared for battle all the time are they not? Or, perhaps . . . (if you're more into nature) . . . :::enter the birds "tweeting":::. . . like a squirrel . . . :)

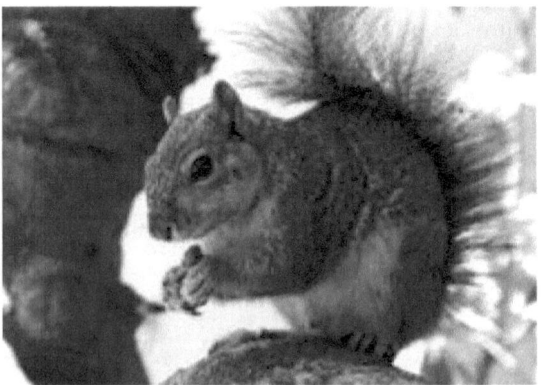

who's gathering and storing for a long cold winter his own healthy food before it is difficult to find any, one should not simply wait for something to come on and not be prepared. No, you have to gather your food (vitamins daily perhaps, please check with your doctor first also) "build your muscles" (exercise, eat organic healthy) and get rid of anything that weakens you (detox maybe, which is so easy . . . see "How to Easily Detox") as much as you can *before* something happens. Here are some "inventory ammo" I try to keep on hand now for my "reinforcements" (*organic* all:) . . .

Braggs apple cider vinegar   Ceylon cinnamon (the best source)
Coconut oil (virgin raw)   Raw honey
Black strap molasses   Garlic
Lemons or lemon juice

and some vitamins . . . A, C1000 (with bioflavanoids and rosehips), B Complex, D3, and Flax seed oil (from as many whole food natural organic sources as I can find).

Look at it this way, if you did simply try it (go organic that is) I'd say for at least a month to give the added hormones, pesticides and antibiotics *(i.e. toxins)* to come out of your system, the only down side? would be is you're *not* giving your body added hormones, pesticides and antibiotics *(toxins)* or any other kind of 'free radical' to combat. You don't have to change any diet you are on! if you're happy with it (i.e. low carb, low fat, low cal) vegan, vegetarian or omnivore. Whatever diet you really feel comfortable with, just use *organic* food in produce, herbs, dairy and meat. My son didn't even think about it until I mentioned one day a few months later how I haven't had to buy as many boxes of tissues anymore (one thing that costs less too by the way). He stopped, looked up from the computer and said "oh yea" :) Now he doesn't need any. So again, it's not something you may see right away. It is kind of "going on faith" in the beginning. I haven't purchased a box of tissues in over two years now.

You should know, I have anything and everything I like *in organic* 'form'. Pizza (hey I'm italian:), burghers with the bun (sorry low carbers:) chicken with the skin (sorry low fatters:) bacon, egg with home fries (sorry low carbers and low fatters:) . . . (yea, this is why I was banished from the *dieters* forum:(. . . 8) Just to add, *yes* I do have vegetables, salads and fruits everyday as well! . . . and I don't have bacon and homefries everyday! I don't have to (though one shared in forum how an old timer attributed his longevity to having bacon everyday!:). I do make my own pizza with organic whole wheat or unbleached flour, organic canned or fresh chopped tomatoes, oregano, garlic and extra virgin olive oil, and mozzarella, all organic. Yes, there is *healthy* pizza after all! So have a healthy organic pizza party! (while you're waiting to lose weight and/or get better) and have some fun! (yep see Rustic's Recipes for my *'healthy' pizza* recipe for that too:)

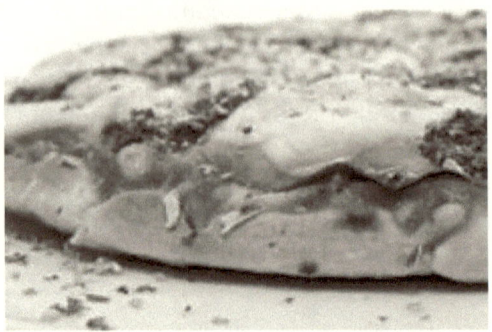

"If we doctors threw all our medicines into the sea, it would be that much better for our patients and that much worse for the fishes." Oliver Wendell Holmes, M.D.

Chapter 5

What do we get?

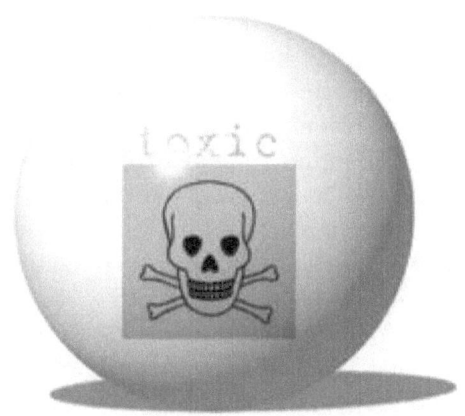

To cure an illness, it would be somewhat important to find out what the actual cause of it is first. That would be the common sense way of doing it anyway in my thinking. Then you'll know from there how to begin to address it right? Whether it be to eliminate the cause in the first place (which would make perfect sense and take priority to me) and then just as important to find the "antidote". And, of course the 'antidote' would have to be or should be something not causing more damage, or the very least as possible at any rate. That would be what "poison control" would have to know wouldn't they. What is the substance first, get rid of it as much as possible, and at the same time apply the safest 'antidote'.

Whenever I try to advocate *organic* food, one of the strange "defenses" (to me) I'd hear is, "Well, organic farms use pesticides too you know!" (?) As far as I can see, one major fungicide is allowed (unfortunately) copper sulfate. (My suggestion is *baking soda*. I wonder if that can be implimented? I used it one time as a *natural* fungicide with water on a new aloe plant very effectively!) Ummm, ok, but *we are* trying to at least have *less* toxins in our food anyway!? That's why we buy *organic*. The USDA actually allows only *certain* pesticides for it to be labeled "organic". In a perfect world, I'd want *no* pesticides, herbicides, fungicides, but, we're the ones advocating for *less at the least?* It's a little puzzling to me as to what kind of argument that is? So, therefore(?) we all should have whatever amount of toxic waste, poison and synthetic chemicals to the heavens (*billions of pounds* each year by the way) used and think they are *just fine* for us and the environment?! It's kind of like an armed bank robber pointing to a child who is stealing a piece of candy, and saying, "Yea but, look what that kid's stealing!" . . . so therefore! . . . see?" And, then of course their very interesting *concern and care* for how much anyone spends on their own organic food. Why that has anything to do with it I'm not sure yet either? I *like* paying more for my organic food! how's that?? :) (please see also my chapter "Consider the Cost" on how you can actually *save* money by going organic anyway! :)

It is true, organic foods are not *necessarily* pesticide-free so I found out (unfortunately). But organic foods are produced using *only certain* pesticides with specific ingredients. Organic pesticides tend to have natural substances like soaps, lime sulfur and hydrogen peroxide as ingredients. Not all natural substances are allowed in organic agriculture; some chemicals like arsenic, strychnine and tobacco dust (nicotine sulfate) are prohibited (used on conventional food though?). You can check the National Pesticide Center online for what is allowed if you wish.

Here's just a few conditions as a result of what we do get in conventionally grown foods . . . I hope you can then decide for yourself if you want to have *more or less?* . . .

Chemicals in non-organic foods can disrupt the endocrine (hormonal) system. The endocrine system influences almost every cell, organ, and function of our bodies (thyroid too) so this is important. It is instrumental in regulating mood, growth and development, and *metabolism*. One type of chemical called *"Obesogens" (Obesogens?! hmmm)* disrupts the function of hormonal systems, leading to weight gain! Obesogens are derived from a variety of sources . . . hormones administered to animals, plastics in some food and drink packaging (BPs), ingredients added to processed foods as well as pesticides, herbicides and fungicides sprayed on produce (designed to kill). In addition, these chemicals *mimic estrogen* in the body. *Estrogen is produced by fat cells, so excessive estrogen causes the body to become more insulin-resistant (where diabetes comes from affecting the pancreas?) and create more fat cells*! Cyclically the fat cells produce more estrogen, causing the body to become more estrogen dominant. More estrogen and more fat cells (from eating sprayed "healthy" fruits and vegetables). Hmmmm

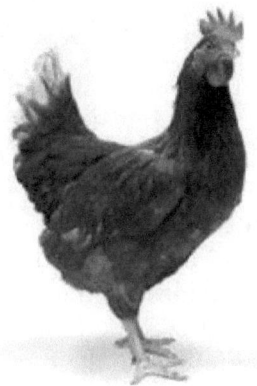

Another thing we may get in conventionally grown and processed foods are *additional antibiotics and hormones (hormones again, always the hormones!)*. Antibiotics and hormones are provided to animals on Concentrated Animal Feeding Operations (or CAFOs) the source of non-organic poultry and meats. The hormones that make the unhappy CAFO animals gain weight faster can also make unhappy people gain weight faster! These hormones are fed to animals to help reduce the waiting time and the amount of feed eaten by the animal before slaughter (as I heard first from my landlord). In dairy cows, hormones such as the recombinant bovine growth hormone (rBHG) are used to increase milk production. Low-level feeding of antibiotics also promotes faster weight gain in animals raised for meat.rBGH is given to dairy cows to make them more productive but it also makes these cows more sickly, causing mastitis (inflammation of the udders, caused by infection) . . . . Ok, so, how is inflammation caused in us then? It is not only cows that are getting sick, rBGH has also been associated with an *increased risk of breast cancer, colon cancer and prostate cancer in humans.* . . Hmmmm. This does mean what the animals are treated with *do* come in us and affect us as well! The additive *has been banned* in Canada, Japan, New Zealand, Australia and the entire European Union—many are calling for a U.S. ban on rBGH, too.

That's not all, antibiotics are given routinely to cattle (and many other livestock) and the drugs show up in the milk the cows produce also. Pesticides too, are also present in the feed of dairy cattle, and these too can show up in milk. The use of these are forbidden in USDA-certified dairy cows, who can only eat certified organic feed (and why it's important to buy organic dairy milk, eggs, butter and cheeses too).

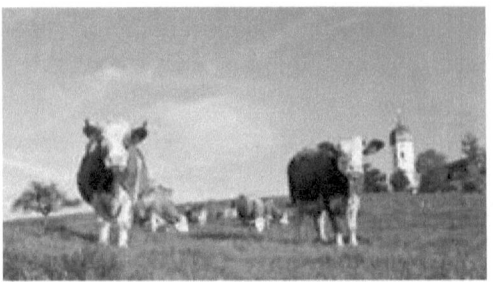

Synthetic Pesticides in U.S.

The use of synthetic pesticides in the US began in the 1930s and became widespread after World War II. Conventional farmers depend on synthetic pesticides to control insects in their crops.

Pesticides have been known to cause lymphoma, leukemia, breast cancer, asthma, and other immune system disorders, hmmmm Again, what is used in and on our food is also being found *in us*. Allergic effects are harmful effects that some people develop in reaction to substances. Why more and more are "lactose intolerant" perhaps? Why more and more have allergies? asthma? My own "hypothesis" is they bring down the immune system and therefore one has allergies. (As my son's allergies left when he went organic also).

Contaminated ground and water (now affecting all environment) *may accumulate in the tissues of animals and be passed up the food chain*, leading to human exposure. Some POPs (Persistent Organic Pollutants) have recently been associated with the *prevalence of diabetes.* (Wait, what's that again? so it's not sugar and diet?) Unfortunately they've been extensively used in the USA since the early 1960s, corresponding to the beginning of the *present obesity epidemic* (yep Hmmmm:).

Fewer Chemicals Needed in Farming Afterall!

I used to consider the reason for non-organic conventional agriculture, and assumed it simply was *a necessity* to use all those chemicals for pesticides and fertilizer because it just wasn't possible otherwise, not on a large scale anyway (so I thought). Then organic farms began to slowly come around, one by one and now we find organic farms *can indeed* produce much more healthy foods with different growing strategies (such as rotating crops also), and with more environmental friendly (therefore better for everyone and everything) pesticides and fertilizers. We *can* grow all the food we need and profitably, with far *fewer chemicals!* It is very much possible! Conventional agriculture can shed much of its chemical use afterall.

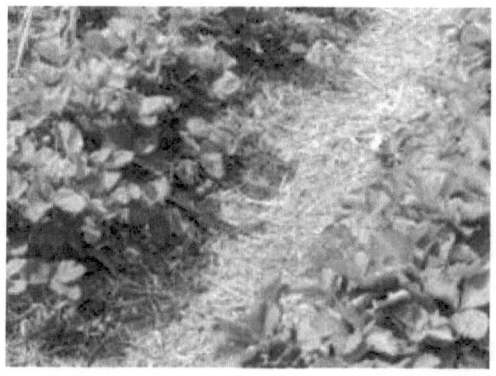

~~~~~~~~~~~~~~~~~~~~~~~~~~~~~~~~~~~~~~

So, what do 'Antibiotics' cause in us?

I mean, in *addition* to keeping us from losing weight? (or causing more weight gain?):/, antibiotics also cause *candidiasis infection* (in both men and women by the way). (Where does illness come from?) I believe most any fungal infection, in the body or on the skin, could be from what we take through foods and meds perhaps? I often wondered, and would sometimes ask the doctor, or on this one occasion the dermatologist, whom I went to see about a rash that I had on my back, what it was? and he surprisingly answered "Candidas". I was kind of puzzled and so I then asked curiously "But, how did I get it?" (not being on antibiotics that I knew of anyway) but he didn't answer. I guess this is my answer? Even if we *don't* take antibiotics in medication, we're still *getting* antibiotics in our supposed *"healthy"* non-organic produced food! And, what do antibiotics cause in us? . . .

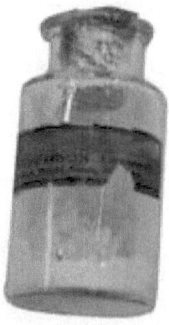

Antibiotic Poisoning Hmmm

Symptoms of "antibiotic poisoning" actually cover a broad range, and the condition can cause a number of diseases from allergies (where do allergies come from?) vaginitis and thrush (that is a whitish fungus in the mouth that actually occurs in babies as well sadly, who get it through the unknowing mother?) to an invasion of the genital-urinary tract (UTIs?), eyes, liver, heart, or central nervous system, wow. And, at it's most destructive, candidiasis is involved in autoimmune diseases such as Addison's disease and Aids.

Here's a list that some alternatives I found have cited:

Gas/bloating, Joint pain, Adrenal/Thyroid Failure, Indigestion, Hemorrhoids, Diarrhea, Ulcers, Constipation, Anti-social behavior (mental illness), colitis, Lethargic/laziness, Heartburn, Suicidal tendencies, Intestinal pain, Dry mouth, Cold/shaky, Depression, PMS symptoms, Infections, Hyperactivity, Irritability, Over & under weight, Headaches, Mal-absorption, Chemical sensitivity, Menstrual problems, No sex drive, Poor memory, Asthma, Epstein Bar Virus, Muscle aches, Skin rash and hives, Diabetes, Colds and flu, Lupus, Burning eyes Respiratory problems, Mood swings, Overall bad feeling, Endometriosis, Hormonal imbalance, Puffy eyes, Dry skin and itching, Vaginal yeast infections, Bladder infections, thrush/Gum receding, Numbness, Premature aging, Finger/ Toenail fungus and Hay fever, wow

Antibiotics kill all bacteria however, that includes the bacteria we do need that keeps candida (antibiotic poisoning) at bay (the same antibiotics sprayed and injected in our foods which we take in every day?). Do you still wonder where sickness and such conditions come from and why they occur? I believe this is why we need more *organically* grown food, for everyone's *health's sake.*

~~~~~~~~~~~~~~~~~~~~~~~~~~~~~~~~~~~

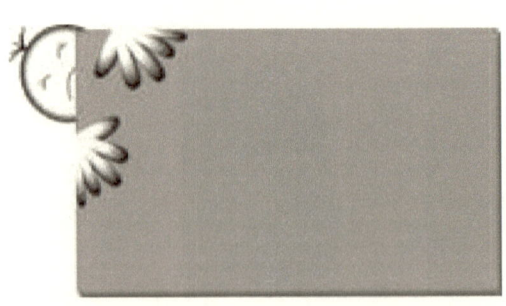

The Bad News

And, how does Conventional Medicine 'remedy' the above?

Ok, the above is pretty much *'bad news'*, but now, notice that most all of those ailments listed are offered even *more antibiotics, steroids, and other artificial substance containing and chemical contaminant drugs* (over-the-counter or prescription) with *more* unnatural ingredients, which then cause *other* areas contaminated with more yeast infections and side effects? So, even though they may remedy or alleviate the symptoms of one? they're actually *causing and/or contributing to another.*

There may no doubt be a place for known conventional medicines but I believe they need to be kept at a bare minimum for instance in an emergency situation? or as a temporary *transitional* treatment if needed. It is amazing the "vicious cycle" it seems we have in conventional foods and medicine together taking in food with toxins causing illness (such as the above) then adding more meds with toxins causing more illness *in other* ways, and so on.

And, What Else Do Toxins Get Us?

Colon cancer is pretty much one of the most "popular" known cancers lately have you noticed? Right up there with prostate and breast cancer. "Get a colonoscopy! . . . soon! . . . regularly! . . ." And, well, pancreatic cancer and pancreatitus (?) seem to be doing some catching up. Did you ever consider why they're getting so *"popular"?* Is it a continuing result of the poor (toxin filled) environment and food supply in our country, and how it is processed? . . .

How Do Meat and Dairy Cause a Toxic Colon? Meat and milk, in their natural states have nutrients, protein, omegas and B vitamins, (we can very much use). The thing is we don't get them in their natural state if they are *not* grass fed organic. Considering the changes that cows go through before they come to us (as described) injected with antibiotics and hormones. They too are *fed* with POP (Persistent Organic Pollutants) sprayed genetically "enhanced" feed. All of which are passed on to humans (you and I) and their adverse affects on our health as well. That would only make common sense to me. You take in 'poison' it will cause bad effects.

When you eat processed foods, these things are part of the process. Rendered gunk are fed to livestock, and your body is called upon to expell what it cannot use. Toxins that come from the food cannot be easily expelled (our bodies are not made for them and become overloaded) and so they remain in the intestinal tract for too long and some are absorbed back into the bloodstream. What remains in the body creates a *toxic colon* and increases the chances of cancer occurring. So where does colon cancer come from? Wouldn't it make sense to *not* take these things in in the first place? Why is that so strange to some I speak to, I still do not know.

"Medicine doesn't get to the root of the trouble. It only conceals it. The result is a more highly poisoned condition which may become chronic disease. All drugs are harmful to the system. They are contrary to nature . . . . Mark my words. There is no way to health except the natural way."

"M," to James Bond 007, in Ian Fleming's Thunderball.

That *organic chocolate cake* seems to sound more and more healthy now doesn't it? :) It's what you *won't* be getting when you *go organic*.

Hormone Disrupting Chemicals in Cleaning Products

A new study by the World Health Organization says a host of common, everyday household products *"pose severe* health problems including cancer, asthma, reduced fertility and even birth defects."

Three *healthy* cleaning products? As you can see, one area to consider seriously also is the household cleaners and other personal products you may use (which would include cosmetics). Three household products for cleaning and room scents, all harmless, very affordable and effective are: Baking Soda, Lemons and White Vinegar. Orange peels, lemon peels, cinnamon and ginger (simmered in water) and some essential oils can be used as air fresheners and scents very nicely. There are also a few new natural and organic mineral products for cosmetics as well to look into.

~~~~~~~~~~~~~~~~~~~~~~~~~~~~~~~~~~~~

The Good News?

So what did I get from Going Organic, taking Vitamins and other natural nutrients?

Alternatives at the very least look for more natural body-friendly remedies. "First do *no* harm" remedies. Some even having other good side *benefits* (I did notice for myself personally). Taking vitamins for some years, and now in particular since going organic, not only has my asthma gotten better? my skin is better too. Even my hands no longer 'chap' in the winter. (The first sign of winter my hands used to dry, chap, swell, itch, get so raw and actually bleed). Being very susceptible to respiratory problems since a child, I haven't had a real cold in over 4 years! (hardly unlikely for me). I do not have high blood pressure or diabetes (both in my family "genes") and "What arthritis"? I barely notice it ever, (except when standing a little too long) and with only my regular calcium with magnesium and Vitamin D supplements thus far. Now since going organic my "borderline" hypothyroidism seems to be turning around (slowly albeit:) heh I do take a natural thyroid complex with iodine and selenium to help my thyroid function better most days.

Something I think unusual is, my eyesight has *not* gotten worse, wearing the same glasses for over 7 years now actually. I *am* eating more organic carrots (now that I'm no longer on low carb) so that may help! :) And, no more heartburn and *indigestion*! And, my sinuses are clearer all without any over-the-counter meds or *any* conventional medicine in years! There are lots of great natural *"do no harm"* remedies out there, and they are the *first* things I would look up if and when I have a problem absolutely. However I just want to make my emphasis here of *at least trying to avoid and eliminate the cause of it all in the first place first!* This is the one thing I noticed some (not all) alternative remedy sites and teachers seem to miss? What is *causing* our illness to *begin with?* and how to *avoid* getting (or at least *stop contributing* to) the ailments (yes even cancer) and most other diseases as well. By *not* taking in the toxins (including carcinogens) and eliminating non-organic food from your diet (as much as you can anyway) back to eating the *real f*oods you were *meant* to have (organic foods) *without the* toxins that *cause* candidiasis and all the rest of the symptoms and illnesses above (whether conventional medicine labels them as *candidiasis* or not *it really doesn't matter* in my thinking*)*. And no, it is *not* snooty or *elitist* to want and have real nutritional organic *(non toxic)* food for myself and my family! :) That is my "hypothesis", and so simply put, here's my prescription:

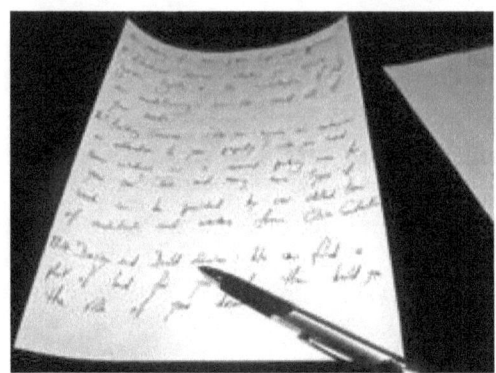

*A: **Detox naturally!*** I started out this chapter with getting to the source of the problem/illness, to which we now can see many are indeed *from* toxins taken in. If we're taking in or are around toxins, then the sensible thing (in my mind anyway) to do would be to detox from them! The following chapter "How to Detox Easily" will give you a few very nice and easy ways to do this.

*B: **Go Organic!*** *(guess I can't say it enough:) heh . . . Prevention!* Really Is the best cure! And so, what is the point of taking in the *cause* again and again, (even after you 'detox') maybe affecting *another* area, and having to remedy over and over? Take yourself out of the 'vicious cycle'. Try to have organic food and filtered water as much as possible! Your body really is an amazing living healing machine, it just needs the *least* toxins to fight off as possible, and it will work better for you.

*C: **Take yur Vitamins!*** Many people may not be getting all the nutrients needed each day (7 to 9 perfectly balanced servings each day?). Try to look up whole food (organic as much as possible) 'First do no harm' vitamins and other nutrient sources for the nutrients you may be lacking for your own particular need (always checking with your doctor first). (See also "Vitamins vs. Vaccines":) If not a supplement then a nutrient rich organic fruit/vegetable powder source might be great too.

*D: **Remedy naturally!*:* There are many "first do no harm" natural remedies I've come across in this last year that I believe are absolutely amazing! Start looking up things like Apple cider vinegar and coconut oil for natural home remedies of all kinds! just for two of them. I've mentioned a few more throughout. I actually came across a testimony of one who used ACV in water each day for his Hepetitis C . . . which he claimed works! . . . so, that's just one other idea to look into.

I would go to conventional methods (for instance in my case an inhaler though I've seen natural asthma mists that I will get to try first if I need it) if and when necessary of course, or in an emergency, or as a *temporary* resort. But, I'm sure even some conventional mds would agree that the less medication and toxins the better? Actually I was told of one not too far from us, whom I may look up when I need to!

***Natural alternative antibiotics* to consider?** Garlic, Coconut oil, Oregano essential oil, Grapefruit seed extract, Collodial silver, High dose vitamin D, High dose vitamin C or High dose Vitamin A.

***Natural* "anti-candidiasas" 'weapons' to have ready?** Yep . . . Apple cider vinegar, Organic Raw Honey, Coconut oil, Baking soda, and Blackstrap Molasses!

Natural Anti-fungals: Grapefruit Seed Extract, D-Limonene (found in oils of citrus), Caprylic Acid a fatty acid derived from coconuts, Probiotics, Olive Leaf Extract, Garlic, Malic Acid (found in apple cider vinegar).

Natural Anti-Inflammatories: Fish oil, GLA, Vitamin E, Vitamin C, all herbs are high in flavanoids which makes them anti-inflammatory, green tea is a good one, turmeric, ginger and olive oil.

~~~~~~

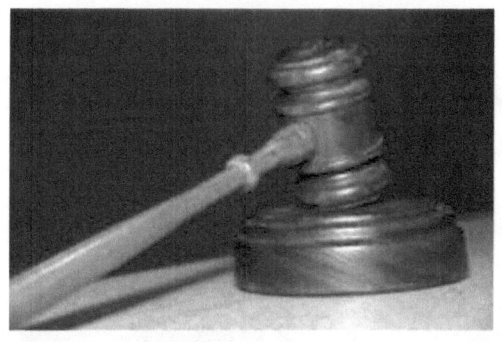

Court Orders FDA to Address Antibiotic Overuse

NEW YORK, N.Y. March 23, 2012 The Food and Drug Administration must act to address the growing human health threats resulting from the overuse of antibiotics in animal feed, according to a federal court ruling issued last night . . .

"For over 35 years FDA has sat idly on the sidelines largely letting the livestock industry police itself," said Avinash Kar, NRDC health attorney. **"In that time, the overuse of antibiotics in healthy animals has skyrocketed—contributing to the rise of antibiotic-resistant bacteria that endanger human health. Today, we take a long overdue step toward ensuring that we preserve these life-saving medicines for those who need them most—people.**

"These drugs are intended to cure disease, not fatten pigs and chickens," Kar said.

The court decision noted, **"In the intervening years, the scientific evidence of the risks to human health from the widespread use of antibiotics in livestock has grown."**

~~~~~~~~~~~~~~~~~~~~~~~~~~~~~~~~

Just a note, if I can't find or buy organic eggs at the time I may look for natural free-range eggs, without hormones and antibiotics (hopefully) in the regular market. You can likely find them in most markets. If you notice, the yoke of the organic free-range eggs are or *should* be a more deeper orange color, (which I am guessing means more Vitamin D?), because the (happy) free—range chickens are getting more sunlight and exercise! yay! Most markets do have organic milk now. Some have organic butter and cream. Mine doesn't, but I just found a place online that will home deliver organic butter, chicken and beef and most other dried items, wherever you live (in the 48 states) so be sure and check to find places that may deliver in your own area as well.

~~~~~~

Vaccines for Everything?

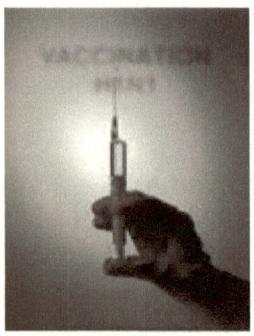

Some things to research for yourself and consider before getting are vaccines. Most vaccines comprise of numerous *heavy metals and chemicals* that may have adverse effects on us as well. (What we need to 'detox' from?). Question the "risk/benefit" ratio always. There is no knowing what nutrient-void chemicals do in other ways even if one does not have initial bad reactions. That would be my consideration in it anyway.

Another issue is, why not have our representatives attempt to address the *root causes* of some disease too (which include filthy animal living conditions and the overuse of synthetic antibiotics in livestock as in CAFOs and as the recent court order stated).

My personal opinion, (the other part of my "hypothesis" here too is) children are simply too deficient in real nutrients everyday, bringing down their immune system and therefore their natural immunity to childhood diseases. Maybe an extra little dose of Vitamin C everyday will help *prevent* a lot of these things alone for them (but please again remember to always consult your doctor).

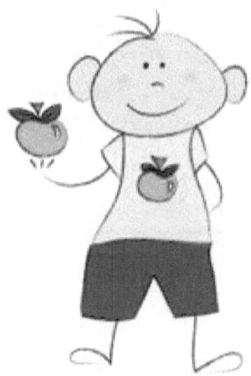

The daily recommendation for a healthy nutritional body strengthening diet to prevent disease is to eat 7-9 servings of fresh fruits and vegetables every day. The problem (in my thinking anyway) is, almost no one does or could do that (except the few posters online that have told me they do so all the time everyday!:). This is where natural whole food supplements may come in. An idea might be to get an organic fruit and vegetable powder mix once again that do have a combination of natural whole fruits and vegetables. You can add them to juice or a smoothie each day without having to buy supplements for the kiddies too. If you look into organic camu camu berry powder as an example, just a 1/4 teaspoon a day provides approximately 500 mg. of Vitamin C alone and easy enough to incorporate into food or drink I would think.

"If we doctors threw all our medicines into the sea, it would be that much better for our patients and that much worse for the fishes." Oliver Wendell Holmes, M.D.

"Let Food be Thy Medicine . . . ."

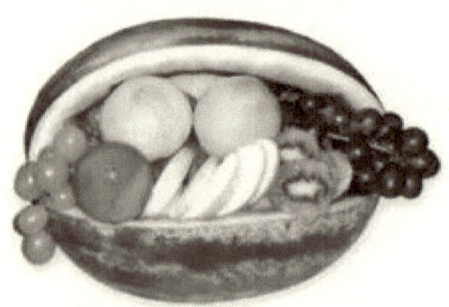

Please remember: Vitamin supplements may have allergy affects in rare cases. Some vitamin supplements may also conflict with any medications you are taking as well. Always consult with your doctor before taking them.

_____

_____

Chapter 6

How to Easily Detox

Learn and live. If you don't, you won't.

U.S. Army training film, WW II

The Good

Now that you've learned of all the *toxins* you've been getting *unawares* in the environment, medicines (over-the-counter or not) processed foods, and perhaps eating with a regular non-organic food diet (though healthy sounding), you probably would like to know now just *how* to rid your body of them effectively and effortlessly? So, here are some things that may help.

The Sun: It is very conflicting and controversial regarding whether the sun is good for you or not I know. Mostly I've heard the sun has to be avoided at all cost?! in the last few years. I saw a dermotologist say how *she did not* want to see anyone with even the slightest suntan. She saw it as being very *unhealthy* and downright *dangerous*. With all due respect, I believe chemical sunblock (if you use it) is more *dangerous* for you, clogging your pores filled with toxins itself. A good rule of thumb to go by is to not injest or *apply anything* on your skin (or your children) that you do not understand what the label of ingredients are! Those are unnatural toxins (i.e. *carcinogens)* that your body cannot process, and everything you put on your skin is going in you *like a sponge*. However, if you are fair skin and do burn easily, that would be the dangerous part. I've read even fair skin can condition to the sun however, by going out in just 20 minute increments so as not to get burned. So, if you must, and you're going to spend hours in the sun, I would consider a very *natural* sunblock, and coconut oil is an ingredient that can be used as a *healthy* one also (I've used it alone and effectively on rashes as an anti-fungal). If you are looking for a healthy sunblock, I found this easy *natural* recipe for you:

3 Tbsp. of shea butter
6 Tbsp. of coconut oil
2 Tbsp of zinc oxide

Put shea butter and coconut oil in a bowl and whisk together. Add zinc oxide and whisk. Zinc oxide is a natural physical sun-blocking agent. Pour the mixture into a container with lid. Apply the natural coconut oil sunscreen to your skin before you head outdoors. Store the unused portion in the refrigerator or the ice cooler (if you're taking it along to the beach). Note: all ingredients can be purchased online.

Coconut oil is a very nice moisturizer alone if you care to use it. Also try it on a fungal rash, or as a deodorant along with baking soda. It might be a note to innovative entrepeneurs or "big corporations" alike (not against free enterprise or big corporations remember) to create a healthy all natural sunblock and other personal items also.

"Sunshine on my shoulder, makes me *happy* . . ."

On the other hand I've heard all the *benefits of the sun!* Please consider the following also: The sun supplies you with natural Vitamin D the sunshine vitamin that actually *prevents* cancer. You get 10,000 to 20,000 IU of vitamin D per hour with no ill effects from the sun in the summer, and with no adverse effects you can supplement with Vit. D3 (the natural D source) up to 10,000 IU daily (which I would consider taking during the winter months especially). Here are some other things to know about the sun:

Getting some sun helps clear up different skin diseases including *acne, boils, athletes foot, diaper rash, psoriasis, and eczema.* The ultraviolet rays in sunshine act as a natural antiseptic. These rays can *kill viruses, bacteria, molds, yeasts, fungi, and mites in air, water, and on different surfaces including your skin.* It stimulates your appetite and improves your digestion, elimination, and *metabolism!* Sunshine enhances your immune system. It increases the number of white blood cells in your blood and it also helps them to be better fighters in their job to destroy germs. Sunshine encourages healthy circulation. It also stimulates the production of more red blood cells which increases the amount of oxygen in your blood. *Sunlight is one of the most effective healing agents that exists* . . . Well, how bad can it be? :)

Basically please use your own common sense. Perhaps use a "healthy" sunblock if you feel you should such as the one given, or look for another, and perhaps "Let *"some"* sunshine in" too :)

Other natural (less controversial hopefully:) ways to Detox?

—Water Fasting

In "It Takes Time" I mentioned my first detox experience actually was an 8 day water fast. Really at the time, I went into it to help lose weight and it did stop the cravings and hunger for a while (which in turn helped me to lose weight). But as I mentioned, I did not know it was the regular non-organic food itself that was causing the cravings and hunger, and contained the things I needed to detox from all along! Water fasting is just one way to 'detox' in any case. If you did, I'd start with one day, maybe 3 days at a time. I would absolutely advise to get a book on water fasting to read up a little on, and help you through if you did. You can actually go up to 40 days max water fasting, to show there is no real harm water fasting a day here and there easily.

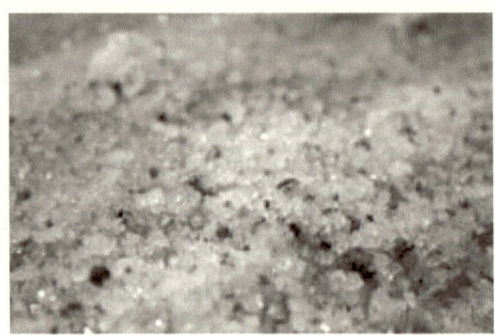

—Sea Salt

When bathing, sea salt gives an antiseptic effect to the skin and reduces histamine that causes inflammation and itching sensation. Sea salt bath can be very efficient in eliminating the toxins of the body while enriching the skin with vital minerals.

—Going Organic!

Simply going organic is *detoxing!* By not taking in the toxins to begin with, it gives your body a better chance to take out any toxins it does have to process, not overloading your liver from doing it's job more effectively.

—Activated Charcoal

Activated charcoal cleanses both the mouth and the digestive tract. Swirl the charcoal in a glass of water and drink it down or mix it with olive oil for easy ingestion by use of a spoon. Activated charcoal is inexpensive, simple to use and is a natural remedy that has many uses without dangerous contradictions, a very efficient cleaner of the body when taken orally. It also helps to purify the blood.

Note: Charcoal may adsorb and inactivate other medications. Usually you can take charcoal two hours before or after other drugs. If you are taking prescription drugs, check with your doctor *before* beginning treatment with charcoal.

You can take charcoal intermittently for long periods or regularly for up to 12 weeks.

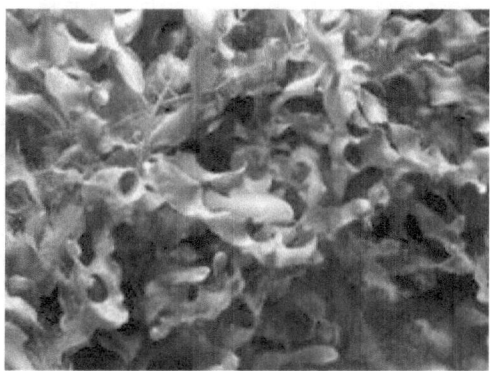

—Spirulina and Chlorella

Spirulina and Chlorella are two supplements we now take daily for a natural source of Vitamin A, but not only that (which is a lot) this is what they also do:

Spirulina and chlorella are two separate micro-algae organisms in the ocean. When taken, they can remove heavy metals from our body from aluminum in deodorant to mercury in dental fillings and metal toxicity. We can try to avoid these substances as much as possible, but some exposure will still occur. Since even *small* amounts of heavy metals in the body can cause negative side effects like fatigue, headaches, digestive problems and skin conditions, it's important to use natural methods to cleanse your body of these toxins also.

—Baking Soda! My New (Old:) Healthy Mineral Hero!

The practice of taking "detoxification baths" is based on the idea of drawing toxins out through the skin during a bath by putting substances in the water that are thought to draw toxins out of the body (remember your skin is like a sponge). Proponents of detoxification recommend ridding the body of toxins taken in through our food and environmental pollution. Baking soda (sodium bicarbonate) provides a naturally alkaline substance helping to remove toxins. Soaking in a bath promotes circulation and the removal of dead skin cells. In addition adding baking soda to your bathwater leaves your skin feeling soft and smooth naturally! I now shower and wash my hair with baking soda and water only. I noticed my hair is less tangled afterwards without any conditioner used. I then may put coconut oil (a little on my hands to lightly rub it in) to help condition if needed.

We use baking soda for many things now including a natural household cleaning product mixed with white vinegar. *Baking soda and salt will clear your drains (recipe below). And, added to some water, I used it to remove a fungus on an aloe plant that was almost totally brown, turned completely green and stayed that way within a day and since! So, baking soda is one item I would always have plenty of on hand!

Those are just a few natural ways you can easily detox with and incorporate in your own healthy lifestyle.

*To clear your drains naturally, put 1/2 cup of baking soda with 1/2 cup of salt (even regular salt this time is fine) on drain area, then pour a pot full of boiling water on them. Repeat a few times if necessary. This has cleared every problem we've had thus far (without any dangerous chemicals).

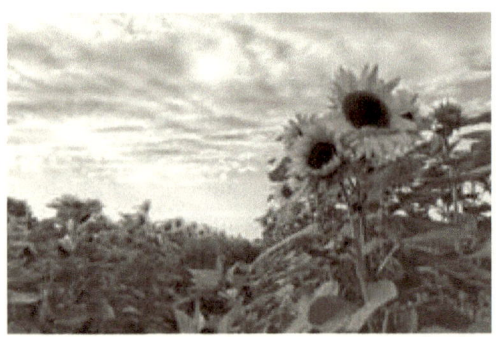

Chapter 7

Just Say No To GMO and CAFO . . .

The Bad :/

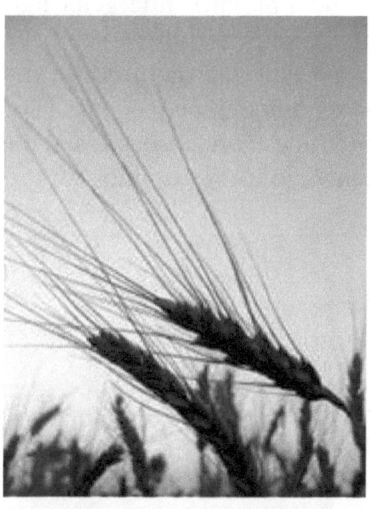

Well you just read "The Good". This is a more and more difficult topic for me as I look into it. I do have a problem with the genetically modified produce (GMO's) the newest form of food production and supposedly "OK" despite no long-term testing on humans taken place. Somehow, (in my mind anyway) if thousands of animals that *were* tested, and their offspring were dropping dead actually having to be *force-fed?* Then I'm thinking maybe they don't belong in us *either?*. :/ That and the fact that they are banned in 30 countries Hmmmm. Just a side note, I also have a problem with microwaves. Sorry everyone! I did read that radiation does *stay in* the foods you "nuke" also changing the molecular value of the food itself. Just thought I'd put that in here since it's used so often for your *wonderful . . . gourmet . . . home cooked . . .* frozen dinners?? Come on people! :) I got rid of mine several years ago anyway, because I didn't want radiation bouncing around the kitchen anymore. Plus! I do *not* believe Chef Ramsey would approve :p :) Maybe try a small convection oven instead? Food tastes better with them anyway!

Back to GMOs :/ I do remember hearing of them a few years back, and remember assuming they would be packaged or labeled as such when I went to the produce section. I really didn't give it much thought for a while since. Like most I'm sure, we're simply too busy to pay attention to what is allowed and we assume our food supply is being looked after safely. The following are some things for you to make your own informed decisions and to perhaps do your *own* research and investigation into:

It turns out, even more chemicals are needed afterall in genetically modified food production :/ There are higher levels of estrogens from "gluphosate" and new and unknown allergens may occur. There may be food and medication interactions and there has been no long-term research to prove safety. There is no labeling required (in the U.S.A.), and unknown and unexpected effects on genetics may occur. There is unexpected higher fat content, and they produce more insect resistence in actuality. *None* of these things are more *beneficial* in my opinion!

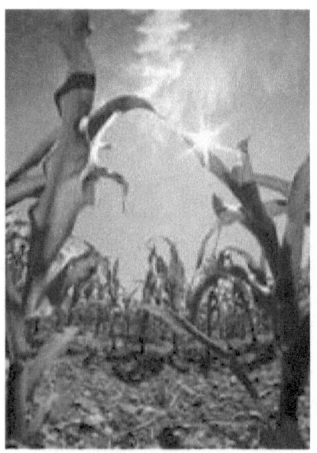

The Sad :(

GM Seeds hurting Indian Farmers and their livlihood: Genetically engineered crops require much more water (which may not be abundant in many places) to grow, and have much higher requirements for fertilizer and pesticides (not good).

Children are most at risk for GMOs: Young, fast developing bodies are influenced most. Children are more susceptible to allergies, and problems with milk, and are more susceptible to nutritional problems. A genetically modified plant could have lower nutritional quality than its counterpart by making nutrients unavailable or indigestible.

Pesticides are now going to be *inside* the food you eat. Considering the increase in illnesses in children and younger people now in their 20's or 30's, I have to wonder how much ill effects gmo's are already taking place.

Environmental Risk: GE crops pose additional environment risks, such as threats to biodiversity or unintentional harm to other insects and animals in the ecosystem, many of which are beneficial to crop production.

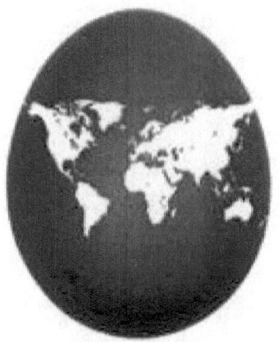

GMOs are Banned Worldwide

Russia and more European countries are now banning GMOs! Japan and South Korea both have recently rejected imports of gmo grown wheat from the U.S., and Hungary has recently burned fields of gmo corn. Those are just the latest that I've heard. Dozens of countries have banned the import, sale, use and planting of Genetically Modified Organisms due to lack of testing and long term study of human health and environmental effects. The following countries have banned or restricted the import, distribution, sale, utilization, field trials and commercial planting of GMO's: Africa: Algeria, Egypt, Sri Lanka, Thailand, China, Japan, Phillipines, Norway, Austria, Germany United Kingdom, Spain, Italy, Greece, France, Luxembourg, Portugal, Brazil, Paraguay, Saudi Arabia.

In North America: Maryland has banned GE (genetically engineered) fish and North Dakota and Montana have filed bans on GE wheat. The Municipalities of Burlington, Vermont (declared a moratorium on GE food), Boulder, Colorado (bans on GE crops) and the City and County of San Francisco (urged the federal government to ban GE food) are the only towns or states to take some sort of stand against plants, animals, foods, crops and body products that are, or contain Genetically Modified Organisms.

The US Does Not Ban GMOs: A conservative estimate concludes that 75% of American foods and body products contain genetically modified organisms. Regardless of dozens of scientific warnings, the FDA has approved widespread use of GMO ingredients in America's foods and body products.

This means almost all non-organic processed foods, (those foods given to our children who are most vulnerable) likely do have genetically modified foods. And when does this get to be animal abuse by the way? No, I am not an animal "activist", and I am not a vegan or vegetarian, but, I do not believe for one moment any animal should be abused like this let alone humans, babies and children. I do believe if most were aware, they'd be against it too.

Tests that have taken place show animals that refuse to eat genetically modified feed, who upon actually being force-fed (this makes me so sad) :(the genetically modified feed develop lesions, abnormalities, disease, and some have died. I saw a clip on a video of a young squirrel who befriended a boy. When the boy gave the young squirrel a 'treat', (it looked like an ordinary cereal square or cracker) the squirrel took it, but then immediately spit it out of his mouth and ran off! My son and I looked at each other, "Was that a gmo??" wow, we laughed but not really funny at all. Animals know and instinctly reject them.

The Ugly :}

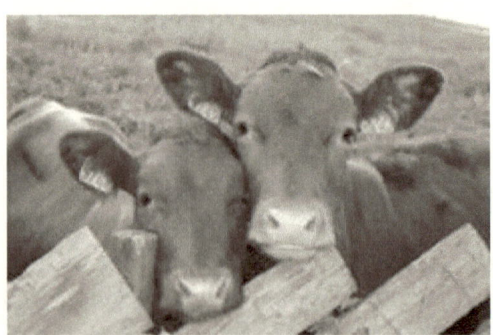

Cafos and Animal Abuse

There is no reason or excuse for the abuse and horrendous conditions of CAFOs (Concentrated Animal Feed Operations). This is really too sad, but I do believe we should all be aware of what's going on today in our food supply, and abusive treatment of any kind.

Cow Concentration Camps: Today it is common for a single feedlot to hold 100,000 animals at a time. Cows are housed indoors year-round. When lactating, most cows are kept tied up in stalls and show signs of stress and the inability to lie down, as well as increased susceptibility to diseases. While corn is the main of cattle feed, many industrial food animals are fed just about anything that can add weight regardless of how unappetizing it may seem. Some commonly used cattle feed additives include poultry feathers, by-products of slaughtered animals, inter-species waste such as swine manure and poultry litter, antibiotic drugs, cement dust, newspaper, and plastic roughage replacements.

Poultry Prisons: The world's tens of billions of meat chickens—"broilers"—grow at an accellerated fast pace. Concentrated in houses with upwards of 20,000 other birds, each full-grown chicken gets less than a square foot of living space. Modern broilers spend their short 7-week lives on top of their own waste encrusted bedding, which the industry refers to as "cake" or "poultry litter," and sometimes enters the food chain as a cattle feed supplement.

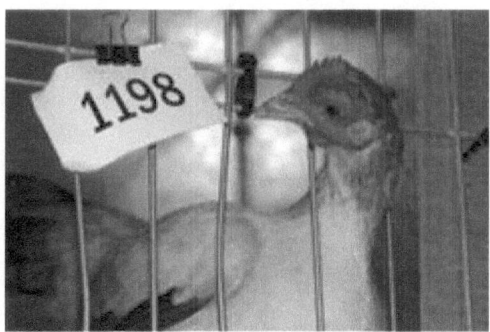

Only USDA-certified organic farms are required to provide *some* access to pasture for grazing. Fewer than three percent of U.S. dairy cows are managed on organic farms.

What Everyday Milk may Contain?: Along with the antibiotics and growth hormones mentioned in "What do we get", 20 painkillers have been found in samples of cow's milk. Even if it's not contaminated, the meat from CAFOs is far from healthy, as the animals have been fed a completely unnatural diet of pesticide-laden GM grains or fishmeal, instead of the pasture or insects they were designed to eat *naturally*.

We are all affected by what's currently happening to our environment and food supply. All those billions of pounds of chemicals, insecticides, waste are going into the ground, water and air as well. I hope the above causes you to stop, think and question what has been happening in our own country, and to consider carefully what is worth putting on your plate. It is not "elitist" or "snooty" to have real food for your own and your family's health and happiness. And, if you want to add to it, how much it will help the environment, the animals themselves, and the earth itself, for us and other generations to come. Simply going organic (though perhaps not *perfect* as some allege and tell me over and over anytime I bring it up :/) it is still a good step in the right direction!

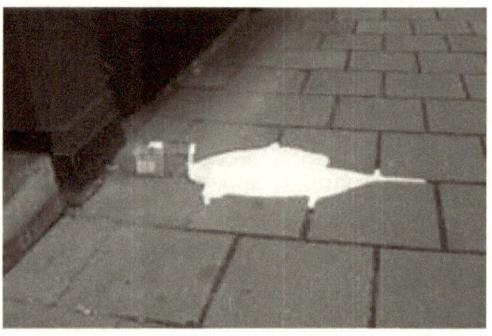

Chapter 8

Consider the Cost

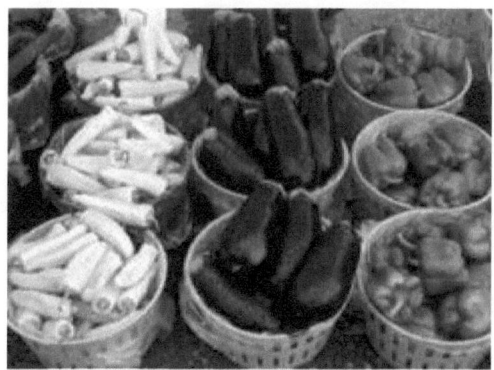

Let's Consider the Cost, *More or Less?*

Ok, now that we got through all of that :/ . . . Let's get to the cost? Yes, I know, organic food is *more* expensive. Trying to be "natural" for some years instead of "organic" I thought "well, it's just too expensive" too. But, then if I think of it, how much more I spent on unhealthy fast-foods, snacks and junk food too. So the cost is offset there for one! Or you might've thought they're for the 'elite' 1%'rs? No, you are just as human, and you need just as real healthy food too! *Say No to GMO and CAFO!* March boldly into your market or health food store and look for *organic r*eal meant-to-be-for-you food. If they're not there, maybe leave a note (if you're too shy) and ask for them. I sometimes leave little stick-em notes around "Organic_____ please, thank you", and I've actually noticed the market near me, and

Walmart's as well, now are carrying more organic! Grocers do listen to the customers.

There are a few other things to take into consideration. If you have a problem battling hunger all day? It will stop, and you will eat *less*. (which will cost less?). Even if you're not gaining weight from it (skinny people do get sick you know?). With my son it was allergies, (which costs less of course not buying all those boxes of tissues), and a skin condition called "backne" also caused by the toxins. That's what acne is actually, toxins coming out of your body. I've heard it has to do with imbalanced hormones, but it's the *toxins that* are *"imbalancing"* your hormones?! In this culture unfortunately young people are taught to cover and mask with even more chemicals (and more money?) to suppress them. If you eat organic foods, and minimize or eliminate chemical household products, it's one good way you won't be taking in (breathing or soaking in) the unnatural chemicals, hormones and antibiotics that may cause and contribute to the conditions in the first place.(And another way to save money too:).

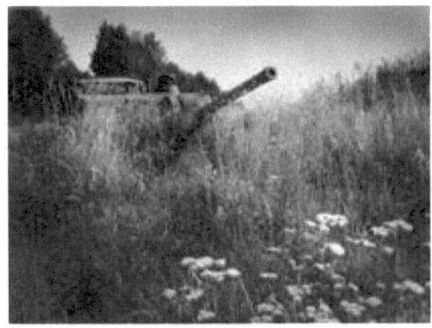

This is War!

Toxins and germs (could this be a kind of *germ warfare* declared on us?) are your enemy. Vitamins, nutrients and non-toxic foods are your ammunition. The fruits and vegetables you will be eating will not be depleted of nutrative value that are used up, trying to cancel out, fight off (*this is war*) the bombardment of 'free radicals' and toxins day in and day out, that you get along with non-organic grown and produced foods. So your body will now be getting *more* of the nutrients and vitamins it actually needs to be healthy too! Your system will be *more* "in tune" again, because you will have *less* "interference" with the unnatural foreign agents and mixed signals it's getting through non-organic grown and processed foods. Your hormones will be *more* in balance *naturally*. Are you really hungry and in need of nutrients or fuel? Or is it the synthetic hormones and antibiotics sending *false signals* to fatten you up too, in the same way they're intended to fatten chickens and cows up? Your body's needs will be *less* confused and more fulfilled.

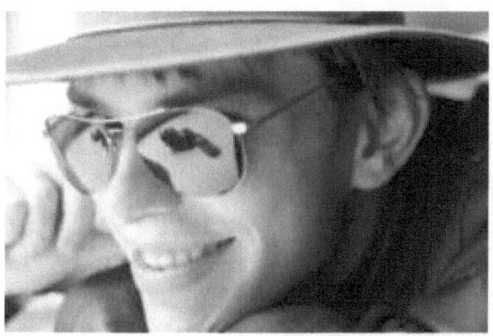

Undercover Agents

I sometimes hear taught how "triggers" to cravings could and *should* be managed by you, and how you can do that in various ways. So how is it that I no longer have these "triggers" and "cravings" I had for so many years that I could barely manage most times? Conventional diets are going on the premise of a regular non-organic diet and foods you're actually *made* to be obsessed over in the first place. You're fighting a confusing (for me, losing) battle against the food you're taking in. Kind of an *"undercover double-agent"* if you will. "Healthful" as they may seem! (yes that non-organic carrot or lettuce or non-fat milk!) but are really *causing* the incessant hunger and triggers themselves, and the battle to eat *less* against it, at the same time taking in the food that's causing it! It is confusing isn't it? When I *stopped taking in* the non-organic foods that were *instigating* hunger ("provocateur"!) . . . I no longer had the constant battle or the confused signals. Simple as that. Those who are into natural health and healing for themselves, are pretty much left to find out most things for themselves it seems, either from our own experience or from someone else's. I'm only hoping my experience will help someone else discover it for themselves too.

A New and Improved *Low Cost and Happy*! "Healthcare Bill"?

Ok, so, one more thing to consider? Your health bill will more than likely *cost less*! Yes! If you are giving your body the *natural real nutrients it needs* eliminating the toxins naturally (undercover agents), your immune system will be stronger to fight off now (with the real "ammo" it's getting) a host of different illnesses and ailments, and you will be sick *less!* Which in turn means *less* dollars on medicines and doctor visits! The last time I had "flu-like symptoms" was only *after* I had a flu shot (which brought down my immune system itself). I haven't had a flu shot since, and *haven't had the flu either.* Amazingly, as I look more and more into this, ailments like asthma, arthritis and allergies also are relatively "a piece of cake" easy to remedy with a healthy natural organic 'living'style, home remedies and real nutrients being more effective now. When you understand that it's *toxins that are the real problem*, and *where they come from*, and what your body really needs to heal and strengthen itself, it becomes clearer who and what the 'enemy' is and posing as like a *"wolf in sheep's clothing".*

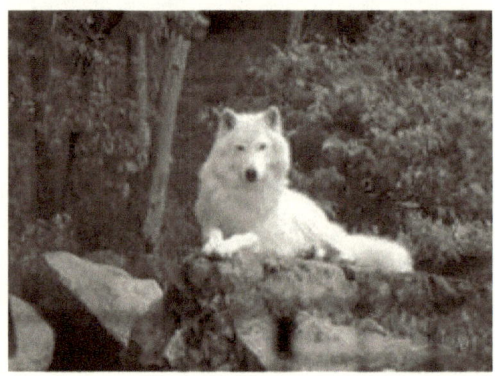

We're actually looking more into things like cancer, how cancer cells are deprived of oxygen by toxins (called carcinogens). It's why we need more *antioxidants (anti-toxidants?)* found in fresh (organic) fruits and vegetables. I just read too one's hypothesis that tumors (at least some) may be the body's response and effort to defend itself from *fungal infection* (candidiasis?) turning in itself. Another is the body being in an too acidic environment, causing *inflammation* as well. It kind of goes together with something else we're learning about, that is getting a more *alkalized* pH balance. And, a *more* alkaline *less* acidic organic diet is what is part of it. So, if we're not taking in the *toxin* filled foods to begin with? *causing* the acidic environment and overgrowth of candidas (from added hormones and antibiotics), our chances *will* be *less* for getting *cancer.* You *are* in control! Right now, our diets are totally thrown off kilt from the start with all the unnatural chemicals and toxins coming into our system, causing cravings for unhealthy foods (whether you're fat or skinny) so the normal amount of food and nutrients needed (vitamins and antioxidants) are far *more* than if we simply had a healthy balanced *organic* food supply and environment to begin with. You will also have to spend *less* time in the supermarket by the way :) having easier decisions to make! Going organic is a 'time saver' as well:)

Six Foods to naturally alkalize and build your defense with: Root Vegetables, Cruciferous Vegetables, Leafy Greens, Garlic, Cayenne Pepper, Lemons

So if you take my suggestion (and "let food be thy medicine") and look up *more* natural ("first, do *no* harm") remedies for most illness and ailments, you will be taking *less* medications, spend *less* time at the doctor's office/hospital? and therefore cost *less* in health care and be more healthy! Basically, you will not only break even *(more or less?)* You'll then . . . be . . . *Happier* and *Healthier* with your ***Awesome! . . . New! . . . Lowcost!* . . . "Healthcare" Bill! . . . Send! . . . Me! . . . to Congress!*** heh :)

*See more *Cost Less, More Healthy* recipes in Rustic's Healthy Recipes section :)

Chapter 9

Drink Water

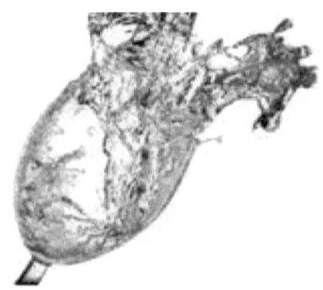

My mom used to have a drink of water, make a face and say *"Ugh . . .
it's Wet!"* and we'd all laugh. Personally it's been the most difficult part of
my 'getting healthy'. OK, that and regular exercise, but, I'm trying ok?! :)
That's another 'vice' of mine, I don't look forward to getting up and jumping
around the living room! but, that's another chapter . . .

Actually, I'm not a 'drinker' at all. I have a cup of organic coffee in
the morning, maybe organic black or green tea (iced in the summer) in the
afternoon or evening, and usually a glass of water with some lemon squeezed
in it with my meals. However, I recently found that I can drink from a bottle
a little better than I can from a cup or glass. Whenever I'd hear I had to
drink 64 oz's of water a day, I'd think, "64 oz's? You've got to be kidding!".
So, if that helps anyone, and you're not a 'drinker' either, maybe you can try
that. Be sure it's a glass bottle (no BPAs). It's easy to keep with you where
ever you go too. Put a little lemon juice in it if you like (organic lemon juice.
If you can't find it in your store, it's on line).

Some benefits of water: keeps you looking young, helps prevent colds
(by washing your hands often) helps you lose weight, cold water splashed

on your face shrinks pores, boosts mood and brain power, lemon in water in morning helps prevent break outs (detoxing), water coming from fruits (like watermelon) and vegetables stays structured long enough to nourish cells in your system with antioxidants (so you can get water that way), a salt in warm water gargle can help a soar throat, cleans naturally (with baking soda, lemon and white vinegar), and the sound of water reduces stress, so get out in nature, next to a brook, water fall, or have a small water fountain set up in your living room perhaps.

Salt: You should know also that if you do not have a high sodium intake, then you do not need as much water. If you do, than you will need more water. Which brings us to the issue of which salt to use too. Celtic Sea Salt is one of the best having natural minerals and nutrients itself. Himalayan Salt (it's pinkish in color) is another. Regular table salt is *not a good thing to use.*

Generic table salt is mined from underground salt deposits and tends to be heavily processed eliminating trace minerals. However, Celtic sea salt (and Himalayan salt as well, we have both) is unprocessed, whole salt. Celtic sea salt is from one of the most pristine coastal regions of France. The water from this region is rich in minerals giving the salt its superior nutrient content and health benefits.

Whether collected from the sea, or salt mines, salt—in its the natural form—is a vital element for all living organisms including essential health benefits. Water, salt and potassium together regulate the water content of the body. Our daily food contains potassium from its natural sources of fruits and vegetables, but not salt (sodium chloride). That's why we need to add healthy salt as celtic sea salt or himalayan salt to our daily diet.

Water Filter: Just an added note, please do use a water filter. They have activated charcoal to filter out many of the chemicals and impurities including chlorine which I used to taste in the water we had from tap. (probably why I never got in the habit of drinking much). My parents had a home upstate also, and when we first went there, and drank the water we thought "wow so this is what water tastes like?!" It was so much more clear and sweeter tasting from the underground water reservoir for the small area, and it made coffee the best!

There is one to filter out fluoride too, as activated charcoal in a regular water filter cannot remove fluoride. (see my commentary "From Fluoride to Freedom" for more on this also)

Fluoride can result in: hyperactivity and/or lethargy, arthritis, lowered thyroid function, lowered IQ, dementia, disrupted immune system, genetic damage, cell death, cancers, deactivated essential enzymes and lower life span :/

Perhaps we should write our officials on how we *don't* want fluoride in our water, and to *please stop 'looking out for us'?!* :)

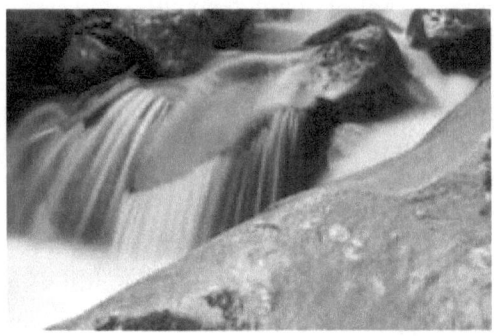

_____
_____

Chapter 10

On To Exercise!

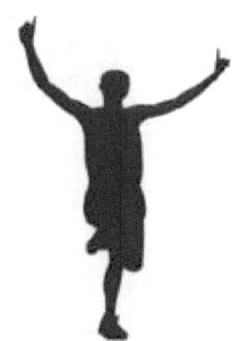

I personally, never understood *'exercise'*. This is the thing, in the beginning man did "exercise" but not in the sense of how we're *supposed* to "exercise" today. Did you ever hear of any 'exercise' regimen in history? No! The man of the household went out hunting (exercise), or tilled the land (exercise), or milked the cows (exercise) or tended the sheep (exercise), chopped wood (exercise) go to war (exer . . . er. :/ :) Okaaay! And the woman? Most likely did all the household chores herself and by hand (of course), washing clothes, spinning wool, making clothes, perhaps did her own gardening, cooking, cleaning, and running around with the children (exercise, exercise, exercise) whew! In other words, they didn't jump around senselessly, walking treadmills, lifting weights, etc . . . etc . . . etc!

Today? me? Well, I get up, get dressed, and walk to my computer and surf :) or hang out in forums and get beat up perhaps with 'negs' *and* *'flagged'!* (that's tiring believe me, dealing with them naysayers) right after making my organic morning coffee with organic sugar and organic milk, that is). That's it! OK so now I try to start some jumping around and some deep breathing (if I am so self-motivated to do so) the very first thing when I wake up! I'm sure everyone is? Right now I do have some fun dvds to exercise with though. I read an article on how just 15 minutes a day of walking will add 3 years to your life! Honestly, I don't know how they could figure things like that out? How *do they* know how long I have scheduled to live to begin with? But, in any case, I'd encourage you to consider it if you do not happen to be into hunting, tilling, spinning, chopping wood, and hand washing your own clothes everyday anyway. I do try to walk to my mailbox a little more often now in the warmer weather too.

Now, before anyone gets out their BMI/BMR charts (or whatever is used now), and how they just *know* that was my problem all along, why I couldn't lose weight? you should know I did do a *lot* of walking, running, and sprinting for buses, walking, running, and sprinting for boats, walking, running, and sprinting for trains, climbing and descending long stairs and long subway corridors, sometimes even jumping! onto train platforms, across flooded curbs or over snow mounds! (Could this be a new olympic event?) Is being pushed and shoved, or hanging on a subway bar or on a bus handle bar being shaken and tossed back and forth at every stop on a crowded bus considered an exercise? (I wonder) for some years working in New York City with an hour and a half one-way commute (and another hour and a half return trip) 5 days a week, an 11 hour work-a-day altogether, and that was on a *good* commute day. (Kind of like a day with Osmin! :/ One time I overheard another passenger ask her friend, "What is this, the commute from *hell?*" and that was her *first* time. Everyone sort of looked at each other, nodding . . . "yep". Then come home to cook, clean, do the dishes and get ready for *the next* day. Ohhhh, yes, my morning started @ 5:30 a.m. with Gilad! and a half hour of . . . yep . . . exercising !!

On the weekends (are you tired yet?) I'd be cooking, cleaning, washing clothes & folding, shopping and walking our german shepherd, **130 lb Bear**, for some extra exercise! (who actually walked me) because I believed I just wasn't getting enough . . . *exercise!* So everyone tells me! But somehow, none of it ever helped me lose weight! No, it was not until I cut out the hormones/antibiotics in non-organic dairy, foods and meat products, and actually went *organic*. I'd say it took me a good two years to sort of *recuperate* from all those years of commuting through New York City and still having to come home and run a household. When I woke up on a beautiful Virginia morning one of the first things that came to mind is "Wow, I don't have to get up, get ready, exercise, walk, run, jump, get shoved, etc etc etc today"! This idea that a woman should be able to do it all? I'd like to tell that person a thing or two or three:) Actually, I believe the best anyone can do (if you don't already have a busy physically active day) is find something you really enjoy, tennis, walking, hiking, skiing, gardening, dancing or whatever else you can think of, that will help you keep interested and active *naturally,* do it and have fun! Kind of that simple in my "unprofessional" opinion anyway, but I'm sure I'm going to hear from all the diet and exercise gurus on this too :)

Chapter 11

My First 'Alternative' Experience

Of several remedies, the physician should choose the least sensational.

Hippocrates

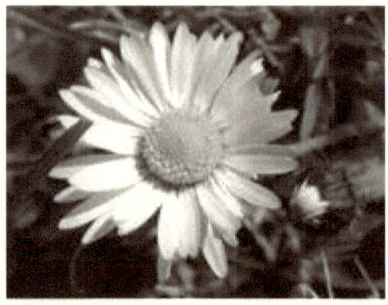

I had an experience as a child, when my throat was closing up after I slept in front of a big fan on a summer night. When I woke up I was all congested and barely able to swallow. If I coughed or tried to clear my throat it would get worse and I'd feel like I was going to choke. My aunt and mom (this was at my aunt's home in Long Island at the time) rushed me to her doctor, who had me lay down on the table, took off my shoe and sock (I remember wondering to myself, "Why is he taking my shoe and sock off? ") and lightly pressed the sole of my foot for one instant. In the next, my throat instantly and completely opened up. That's the best I can recall and without any exaggeration. I only remember one other thing, him bending down looking at me with a smile afterwards, asking "Are you ok now?" I just nodded yes slowly, kind of puzzled though. lol Nice looking young doctor too.

Now, I know you're not going to believe that one too easily, and I totally understand! I'm not too sure if I believe it myself now. I was maybe 5 or 6 at the time. I can image it pretty clearly though, being one of those clear unforgettable memories, and somehow I image it was my right foot. It was never spoken of (to me anyway) after that, I was kind of young, and I didn't look into it for a long time of course, and I never brought it up to anyone else. It was just "one of those things". But then years later I'd hear a little from time to time having to do with nerves connecting to different parts of the body called "acupressure". I still don't know much about it, but thankfully nothing else had to be done. Now my wondering is, what if the medical profession did open more to "alternative" remedies and procedures like that all these years? Imagine what the ER would look like today? That doctor, fortunately for me, was ahead of his time.

Of course I don't dismiss today's technology. Well, except when it comes to internal medicine. I believe our bodies were not created to handle non-organic chemicals that well. Yes, I would take *emergency medication and/or anesthesia* if I should ever be in an accident, or something of that sort, as one in the health forums tried cornering me on. It's just that we have *living* bodies, that need *living* nutrients, and I would try to keep it to a bare minimum. Yes, I would take my inhaler again, if I had to! but I would then continue to look for other natural homeopathic remedies in the meantime. That's the best way I can put it. It's still strange to me how *defensive* some are of chemicals *poisons and toxins!* So, they would not accept what that doctor did to help clear my throat? because it's not conventional medicine? Would they, if they were in that situation turn down the treatment? I'm sure they wouldn't.

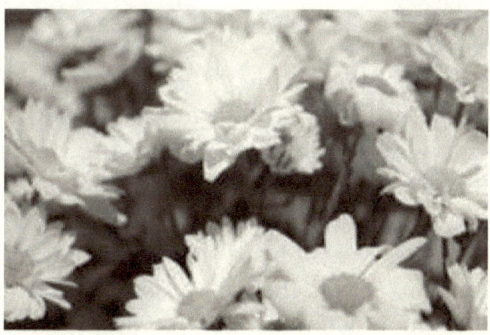

Chapter 12

It's a "LivingStyle"

Without health there is no happiness. An attention to health, then, should take the place of every other object. Thomas Jefferson, 1787 (b. 1743-1826)

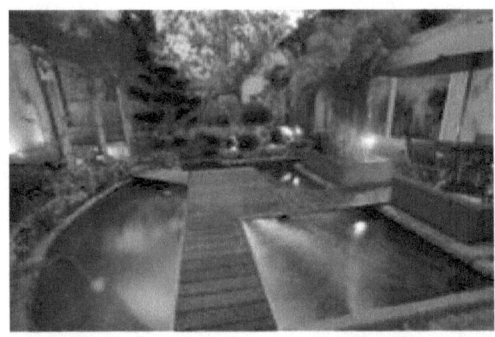

Getting healthy is a 'living' style. I use as much natural and organic products as I can now in order to hold down synthetic toxins in my life. By eliminating as many as possible you're allowing your body to build your 'immune system' from within to fight off "intrusions" (free radicals and toxins) from without, in all different ways. I have to say, that if nutrients and a healthy organic diet has affected the outward symptoms I've had and mentioned? *then I have to believe* they are *absolutely* helping things we don't see like heart health, like blood pressure, like diabetes, like . . . *Cancer*.

A mammogram showed a small lump several years ago. I also had an ultrasound and saw the the small "lump" for myself. I was supposed to make an appointment for a biopsy ASAP! Thinking as I went up to the lobby, looking over at and passing the "appointment desk", I walked slowly . . . to my car . . . and went home instead. I didn't personally want to go through the ordeal of testing and/or recovery and such. Some say it's nothing (a biopsy) but, at the time I had heard some not so easy things. Actually, it took a while for me to get that first mammogram (and that was enough pain for me). I decided to increase my vitamins and continue to eat healthy instead. I believe I heard even if you *are* treated and cured, five years later it may or may not come back anyway. I thought I'd rather do my best at the least feeling good for five more years if I could. This was about 8 or 9 years ago.

I know it was a risk, but that's the risk I personally was willing to take. I went back six months later for another mammogram and ultrasound, and after what seemed to me to be a very long wait of another results, the nurse finally came out with a smile . . . "We can not find the "lump", nothing is showing" (or something to that effect, I don't remember precisely, it was kind of too tense for me at that point and I was kind of in shock). I remember looking at her a little disbelieving. It did take so long for her to come out that I began pacing . . . worrying . . . *"Now you've done it Patti"* really assuming the worst. Now, I was told that that *has* happened before. I did see the "lump" myself in the ultrasound screen (about a dime size) so I'm not sure where it went either, or whether it was my vitamin and healthy eating regimen that had anything to do with it, but, there it is and here I am! Please understand I am not telling *anyone not* to get a biopsy! One "concerned" troll :) plastered this incident (when my site was for anyone to see) in a health forum to showcase my "ignorance" of not getting a biopsy I suppose (and my illiteracy:) not being a writer, only blogging my experience at the time) I would absolutely suggest you do get one if it is called for! What I am saying is to please keep in mind I had for some years already been taking a number of *vitamins* (especially Vitamin C in my opinion anyway) so, in that sense, what I'm really trying to say here is . . . *why wait* to the point of having a "lump" or any other condition or illness *before* changing your 'livingstyle'? Very few are getting enough vitamins and nutrients I believe (in perfect 9 serving a day meals)! If that were so, why are we still getting sick? (besides the reason of too many toxins that is?). Wouldn't that be the indicator that we're *not* getting sufficient nutritionally filled diet all the time? Why not make it your *livingstyle* to help *prevent* or perhaps *lessen* any impact of illness in the future is what I wish to convey here. And, by the way, if I had to get a biopsy again, (hopefully it's as easy as they claim) and I did find out I had cancer? I'd be very happy and relieved to know there are other things that can be done to help anyway! such as . . .

Vitamin D Linked with Smaller Tumors

Women who have higher levels of vitamin D when they are diagnosed with breast cancer appear to have smaller tumors, according to a new study. When I had my mammogram done nothing was said about Vitamin D deficiency at the time. Hopefully they are prescribed more to women now! (D3 is the natural source, D2 is the synthetic composition)

Benefits of Vitamin D

Maintains Calcium Balance
Aids in cell differentiation
Boosts Immunity
Blood Pressure Regulator
Aids in Osteoporosis
Alzheimers
Autoimmunity
Cancer

I now take 5000 mg of Vit D3 per day, however, I understand 10-20,000 mg is not too much.

Of course I am not saying I've achieved *perfect health*, or will never ever get sick again! That's silly. My bp is 130/70 right now. Guess I'll have to have more dark chocolate!:) Of course I will still have problems. I've had a lot of years of 'abuse' (being attacked by all kinds of "free radicals") so I still don't know what may or may not be brewing or if I caught them 'free radicals' in time or not? but what I am saying here is, I've had enough evidence for myself so that if and when I do have a problem? I will absolutely look into my own diet, what foods to eat for what and natural *"first, do no harm"* remedies, herbs and vitamins, if I should need them first and foremost. The internet thankfully is absolutely great to look up and find many things like this . . .

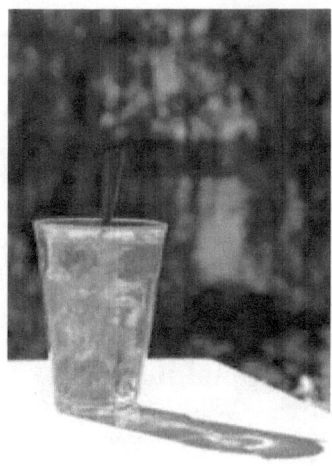

Green Tea Cancer Crusher?

Green tea may help protect lungs better than black tea does because green tea has more cancer-fighting antioxidants called *catechins.* And green tea catechins appear to thwart cancer in myriad ways. Lab studies show that a special kind of green tea catechin called "epigallocatechin gallate" may slow the growth of human cancer cells and may even trigger their death! Yes! Other green tea catechins are great at neutralizing cell-damaging free radicals that open the door to the cancer process.

The great news is, it's your *livingstyle* (not your genes) that will determine your own health! You have the ability to change your own condition. It's not simply "written in your genes". You can alter them on a regular basis, depending on the foods you eat, the air you breathe and the water you drink. Try drinking more green tea for instance! I may drink it more now too, hot in the winter and iced in the summer.

Foods that also help fight Cancer?

	Turmeric	Carrots	
Cabbage & Broccoli			
	Tomato	Garlic	
Flax seeds			
	Blueberries	Hot Peppers	Green Tea
	Broccoli	Pomegranates	

The Cottage Cheese and Flax seed oil Diet and Lung Cancer

My son showed me this one who responded to one of his own posts on youtube . . .

"My dad was diagnosed with stage 3 lung cancer about a year ago . . . He was 79 at the time and did not want any form of treatment . . . I started him on the cottage cheese and flax oil and some of the cancer has shrunk and has not spread . . . He is stable with no coughing, good appetite and has been getting good reports . . . He does this 2x per day and so far so good . . . We feel it's better than nothing and the doctor just shakes his head in awe when he sees him . . . ."

The flaxseed oil and cottage cheese protocol can be found on livestrong. com as well as other sites by the way. It also called the "Budwig Diet".

Baking Soda, Molasses and Stage 4 Prostate Cancer

Another experience I came across is one who used baking soda and molasses to actually cure his stage 4 prostate cancer! He was told to go home and that there was nothing else to do at the time. However, his son told him to look up "pH and cancer" on the internet. From that he purchased some baking soda which alkalizes bringing down the acidity in the body, (fighting inflammation?) mixed it with molasses and water, and drank that each day. A few years later and he's fine! The premise is that cancer is attracted to the sugar in the molasses, but mixed with the baking soda, the baking soda then "attacks" the cancerous cells and destroys them! Kind of a "trojan horse". So, if you wish to, you can look that up on the internet for more specifics. This man's website is *www.phkillscancer. com*.

—

In case you were wondering if the baking soda and molasses protocol helps prostate cancer only? (well I was wondering anyway:) two more wrote on the above site of their own experiences. One with pancreatic cancer, and in a lot of pain. Did the baking soda and molasses protocol, and a few days later woke up with no more pain! . . . another wrote of his father's renal cancer also, and for 2 weeks nightly did the protocol and has noticed huge improvements . . . being able to walk, eat and think better than before! Those are amazing to me! So it's not only for prostate cancer which is great to know also.

It should be noted also that the site above advocates maintainance of an *alkaline diet: at* least 80% Alkaline and 20% Acidic. A comprehensive list of alkaline/acidic foods can be found at http://rense.com/1.mpicons/acidalka.htm.

There are hundreds of thousands of other testimonies people write about also (not only with cancer), and another great place to look up some of those ideas and personal "anecdotal" experiences is EarthClinic.com.

Inflammation and Cancer

One brought up an article of how *"inflammation"* is a cause of cancer recently. Chronic inflammation is a "complex prolonged internal response to a tissue insult". This response involves the immune and endocrine systems. Well, you know what my theory would be? put simply, inflammation caused from yep, *Toxins . . .* just like heartburn? Well, in any case, I would then look up anti-inflammatories in food sources to have as well as take in as least toxins (inflammatories) and non-organic foods as possible!

Some Anti-Inflammatory foods? Cold water fish, green tea, turmeric and ginger, vegetables, fruits and olive oil.

Anti-Inflammatory nutrients? Fish oils, GLA, Vitamin E, Vitamin C, MSM, Flavanoids, and Botanicals.

So, What Is the "Rustic Cure" for Cancer?

In the beginning of the book I spoke of help in all kinds of illness and ailments set upon us, and I stated what seemed to me to be the 7 major and prevalent "diseases" today: Asthma, Arthritis, Allergies, HBP, Heart Disease, Diabetes and *Cancer.* And yes I remember asking . . . ."*Even stage IV Cancer??" in the first opening paragraph.* Well the above give just a few possibilities that I would certainly look into and try personally! Baking soda, molasses, flax oil, cottage cheese? What can hurt?? What would be the harm?? in particular at that stage? I'm not sure why anyone would want to suppress anyone from making their own choices in health in anycase. That's a personal decision isn't it? It's kind of strange to me indeed. But, on a larger scale, this would be my prescription and "cure" for *all kinds* of *Cancers:*

Eliminate** the **Carcinogens** that are **Causing** the **Cancers! Found in our food, water and air now, (*Billions of pounds per year?)* of pesticides and all kinds of *cancer causing* chemicals, hormones and antibiotics that cause the fungal infections (if that indeed is what some cancers are, an overgrowth of candidas and the body's effort to turn in on it and protect itself) and the *inflammation,* as stated above (that seems to be part of a few other conditions like arthritis, fibromyalgia, etc.). This could and should be done on a large scale obviously, limiting drastically what is allowed to be used in production of all of our foods just for one, which in turn affects our own water supply as well. (Perhaps writing our congressmen to address this afterall?).

And, on a personal level?

Detox easily . . . once again consider some of the natural detoxing methods in Chapter 6 **"How to easily Detox"**. *And, **Stop taking in the Carcinogens!*** one way being to ***Go Organic*** :) as much as possible of course, and also eliminate as much around you in household cleaning products, and personal items as well, such as soaps, moisturizers, sunblocks and cosmetics. And, yes . . .

Take yur Vitamins! I've been taking *Vitamin C* all these years to help my asthma, (which it did terrifically), but had no idea what else it actually may have been benefitting? One of them is it helps take heavy metals and toxins (i.e. carcinogens) out the body! So, if you're not getting all the Vitamin C you may need in natural whole food fruits and vegetables, then that may be an option to help (and look up kamu kamu berry also). Vitamin D is another (and get some sun!). And of course there are others, herbs like green tea stated above, so, those I would personally consider also.

As in war, one would go at the enemy from all angles, and those are the few I would do in going against the *cancer enemy* as well! I don't believe or would limit it to only one particular formular, pill or procedure. That would be the "Rustic Cure" for cancer! I state pensively awaiting the imminent "law suits". :)

A "Rustic" thought on Inflammation and Alkalizing

So, what do arthritis, addison's, alzheimers, acne, autoimmune diseases, celiac disease, chronic prostatitis, cholitis, chrohns, dermatitis, hepatitis, IBS, lupus, parkinson's, rheumatoid arthritis, ulcerative colitis (and a few others) have in common? They're all chronic "inflammatory" diseases.

Inflammation is the body's natural process of healing. However, an *excessive* amount of inflammation results in chronic ailments (as listed above). Do unnatural chemical substances coming into the body *cause* the inflammation as well? That would be something to consider also. So, wouldn't going organic (not taking in the chemical "inflammatory" substances) help stop the cause of inflammation occurring? and therefore ease some of these diseases. Well, you know my consideration would be "yes" it would, and it would help to cut down on them very much!

Regarding "alkalizing"? In chapter 2 I shared a little of how a woman was healed of her crippling arthritis by taking apple cider vinegar and honey! I also shared how I took calcium with magnesium for my own arthritis and have had no real problem in years. That struck me as curious for a long while now. What could apple cider vinegar, honey, calcium and magnesium have in common to ease arthritis? Now, one thing I've been looking into lately is "alkalizing", and what foods and nutrients do that. And lo, and behold?! what do calcium, magnesium, apple cider vinegar and honey have in common? They are all *alkalizing!* They are all beneficial in fighting *inflammation!* And arthritis is a chronic "inflammatory" disease! So, that's a huge thing in my mind, and to keep in mind when looking for help in some of these other chronic inflammatory diseases as well. Anyway, just another "blithering" rustic thought :)

Please Note: a comprehensive list of alkalizing foods and nutrients can be found at: http://rense.com/1.mpicons/acidalka.htm

A better way to detect cancer? "Thermogram's" specifically measure *inflammation* . . . hmmmm A poster put this up just recently:

"Thermol imaging" or "Thermography" is the newest state of the art non invasive safe diagnostic tool that can test for cancer and many other conditions long before a tumor mass is detectable by conventional mammogram. Thermography is inexpensive quick safe simple and you recieve NO RADIATION EXPOSURE . Thermography is able to detect tumors the size of a grain of rice that would go unnoticed on a mammogram.

Thermography Diagnostics Center at 847-252-4311

Natural Ways with Depression

Just to touch upon it, I believe not all perhaps, but many mental illnesses may be caused by yes toxins and/or nutrient deficiency! I have no way *of proving* it of course, I just think it's possible, and why some may be fine, but then unexpected, unexplained, or after having some kind of drug, have a kind of break down. In any case, I would consider nutrients and detoxing as something to consider and try also. Here are a few safe and effective ways to address depression without unsafe drugs . . .

Decrease consumption of sugar and processed foods (I did this naturally by going organic very easily remember). Increase *consumption of probiotic* foods such as fermented vegetables. Get adequate *vitamin B12*. Optimize *Vitamin D levels* . . . (get some Sun!) Get plenty of *omega 3 fats*. The brain is 60% fat, and (grassfed) *animal based omega 3 fats* are crucial for brain function and mental health. Adequate exercise, and adequate sleep. For difficulty in sleep increase melatonin (found in oatmeal for one).

Organic Grass Fed Beef High in Nutrients and *Omega 3s*

Beef in Australia contains high levels of nutrients, including the omega-3 fatty acids that are important to mental and physical health. This is because cattle and sheep in Australia are largely grass-fed. In many other countries, the cattle are kept in feedlots (CAFOS) and fed grains, rather than grass. This results in a much less healthy meat with more saturated fat and fewer healthy fats (with omega 3's). I have found a few that are here in America so please look locally or online for one that may deliver to you also.

Whole Grains rather than statin drugs to bring down cholesterol?

Regarding cholesterol, my own experience is having a bowl of oatmeal everyday for a month or so brought down my own cholesterol. My doctor thought it was amusing when I told her what I did, but, it worked! I pretty much have it and other organic whole grains every day now . . . when in discussion on a health forum this is what someone there said . . . **crystbear (my old nic), I'm with you <********>**

I couldn't take statin drugs, so I did the whole grain breads and cereals, I dropped my LDL over 150 points and raised my HDL by over 50 points.

Just personal experience.

There is always a more natural safer way of health and healing and *'livingstyle'* in my opinion.

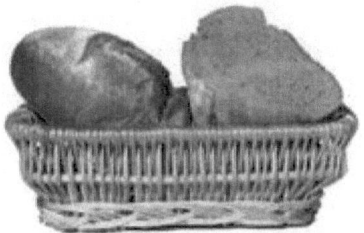

"If we doctors threw all our medicines into the sea, it would be that much better for our patients and that much worse for the fishes." Oliver Wendell Holmes, M.D.

Chapter 13

My Own Happy Conclusion

He who lives by rule and wholesome diet is a physician to himself. from: Concise Directions on the Nature of our Common Food so far as it tends to Promote or Injure Health. Published by Swords of London: 1790, p 7.

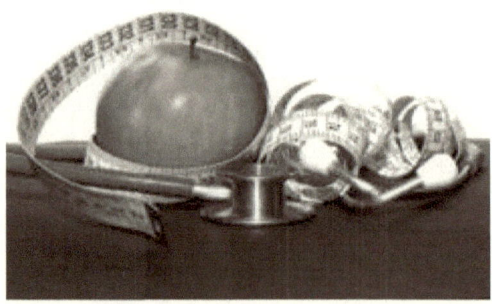

I'm kind of sure you have felt helpless about illnesses and such from time to time, just as I have. Have you wondered if or when *'cancer'* may come and get you or one of your loved ones? My own younger brother died (and went to heaven) at the age of 28 of hodgekins disease so I know how difficult it is. Or how complicated everything seems. Certainly it would take those very very educated to figure it all out! Or many more years (though they keep saying there's a "cure" coming right around the bend!) *and billions* more in cost for research and taxes :/ Well, I'm here to tell you it's not true, it's not true at all. It can actually be amazingly affordable true low cost and effective healthcare, and happily simple too. Remember to find the source? I hope I've encouraged you to seek out natural and safe remedies on your own, *"Be your own doctor"*, for you and your family's sake. I don't doubt that most young people start out going into the medical profession because they really want to help people, and they still do. It's just what is taught (and omitted perhaps) in the educational institutions, that seem to be a problem.

Here's another example of what one shares regarding her kidney stones . . .

****: **"I have suffered intermittently from kidney stones for nearly 9 years. One was so bad I had to have surgery to remove it. Later, my grandmother was hospitalized with a kidney stone and told me about a home remedy given to her by a nurse and believe me, this really works! *Mix 2 oz of olive oil and 2 oz of lemon juice, drink it straight down and follow with a large glass of water at the first sign of stone pain. The stone(s) will pass within 24 hours. I have eliminated at least 8 stones with this remedy and have not gone back to the urologist since I started taking this."**

I have shared my own personal "anecdotal" experience, experiments, and opinions here (and quite a few of others) and the little I've learned mostly in this past year, and what has worked for *me* thus far. I may change things for myself as I am still learning as I go! (being my own doctor). But, one thing I know, whatever *'diet'* :p I may choose? since I still have some losing to go (if any:) it will be with *organic real foods*! Or maybe I'll try that 3 apples a day:) I believe a holistic doctor can tell you a lot more and explain things a lot better. If you haven't already checked them out, there are a few on the internet and have written books that I've found very informative and helpful.

We're told regular produce have as much nutrients as do organic. But, even if that were true, (which I still find hard to believe) the added poisons and pesticides (toxins) are still something you will be dealing with and are the cause to begin with of almost all illness and ailments. Fighting, healing disease and ailments while continuing to contribute what is *causing* them (remember the undercover double agents) does not make sense to me! So, *"Let food be thy medicine, and medicine be thy food"*.

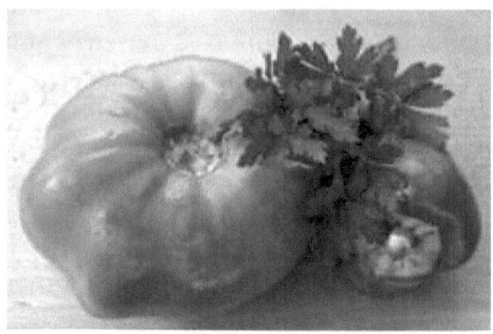

Naturally I would say use *organic* foods whenever possible. I've listed here however, the 14 regular produce you can buy that are not laden with pesticides for you to bring to the store or market with you when you go to help keep down the cost . . . Or hey! Grow your own! . . . I plan on doing it perhaps this spring starting with a few containers.

"Organic gardening is not just the avoidance of chemicals, in the larger view, it is organic living using nature's laws".

Onions	Pineapples	Avocados		
Asparagus	Kiwi			
Sweet Peas	Mangoes	Eggplant		
Cantaloupe (domestic)				
Cabbage	Watermelon	Sweet Potatoes	Grapefruit	
Mushrooms				

12 produce called the "dirty dozen":

These are the produce most containing or sprayed with pesticides and antibiotics as above:

Non organic peaches	apples	sweet bell peppers	celery	nectarines
strawberries cherries,	kale	lettuce		
imported grapes	carrots	pears		

I only buy them if and when they come *organic.* A site you can check out most any different produce is *www.whatsonmyfood.com* to see for yourself and compare to regular foods and produce as well.

My only wish is you also will look into some of these things I've shared here, find a little hope, (actually, find a lot of hope)! if you think *it is 'hopeless',* or that you are helpless; even if, and especially if, you have something serious. *Be positive, be proactive,* (get plenty of "ammo") so that you too will be happy getting healthy too.

Patti aka: crystbear, now: *RusticHealthy! :)*

"If we doctors threw all our medicines into the sea, it would be that much better for our patients and that much worse for the fishes." Oliver Wendell Holmes, M.D.

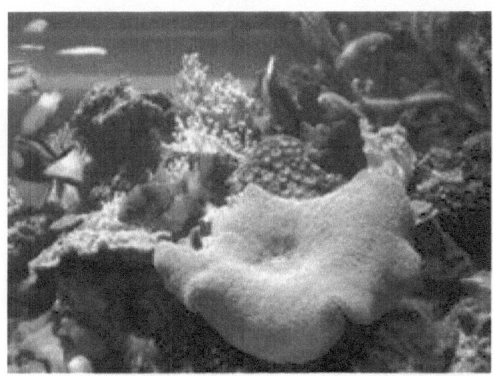

Information and accounts written here and throughout this book are for entertainment, anecdotal, and not intended as a substitute for the advice provided by your physician or other healthcare or holistic professional. You should not use the information for diagnosing or treating a health problem or disease, or prescribing any medication or other treatment.

Please remember: Vitamin supplements may have allergy affects in rare cases. Some vitamin supplements may also conflict with any medications you are taking as well. Always consult with your doctor before taking them.

Rustic's Healthy Commentaries

These "Rustic Commentaries" were written throughout the year, with a little more information in my searching and surfing, and some of what I've personally encountered. :)

*   *   *

Rustic Commentary 1

My Hypothyroidism

March 2012

This is my first "Rustic Commentary" here, and so I'm starting with what's been a big part of my experience (i.e. weight battle :/) all these years, having "borderline hypothyroidism". Some years ago I was told I was 'borderline' having a difficult time losing weight, and the doctor wanted to give me a mild medication (for the rest of my life). I just didn't see it as that big of a problem then, and didn't like medications anyway especially to have to stay on "forever", so I decided against it. This was before too much was said or known about hypothyroidism (that I heard of anyway). Most of the time it was considered an *"excuse"* for someone having a weight problem if it were ever mentioned. I kind of totally forgot about it as the years went, and continually tried fighting it and dieting on my own. Taking vitamins appears to, or I believe has been a good thing I did in the meantime. Having "borderline hypothyroidism" does explain a little of why I could not lose weight easily, and keep it off as well. As mentioned in "What do we get?" my belief is it's because non-organic foods shot up with hormones, antibiotics, or sprayed and grown with chemical fertilizers, pesticides and so on, affecting the *thyroid* (metabolism) along with most everything else in the body.

Now since going organic, it seems to be reversing slowly, losing weight a little more easily (and keeping it off importantly no longer on a roller coaster) and having fewer symptoms. I am now taking iodine, in the form of kelp supplements, and a thyroid complex with selenium and other things. Vitamin D3 is important for hypothyroid, and I am taking that now also. I tested 27, which indicates I am on the right track dealing with it so that's good news! Still slow losing weight, but at the least not roller coastering and gaining more as I did all these years! If you go to this site, WomentoWomen. com, and take the test, you may be able to see for yourself if this is your problem as well. I am going to follow some of the ideas given on it, (or not:) what foods to have and how they should be cooked, but always *organic!*

If you are already on Thyroid medicine, this is a site to learn some important things . . . *www.stopthethyroidmadness.com*

And, if you're not on thyroid meds, here is a good site to find out what you can do alternatively . . . *www.healthwyze.org/index.php/component/ content/article/211-curing-hypothyroidism.htmlOne*

Coconut Oil for Hypothyroidism?

One compelling testimony regarding **hypothyroidism and coconut oil!** (my new oil favorite) . . .

[] : . . . . **"My Dr. wanted to put me on synthroid. I asked how long I would need to be on it. She told me, for the rest of your life!!! I said there must be a natural cure. She said no. I wasn't convinced because I had heard from my mom (who is a nutritionist) that the body is designed to heal itself. Those words always stuck with me.**

So I did research on my own and found that coconut oil was what I needed to get my thyroid back to normal. So I tried it. 1 TBSP per day for the 1st week, 2 TBSP per day the 2nd week, then 3 the 3rd week. I saw my Dr. at the 3 week mark and was tested again. My TSH level had dropped to 7.8. Dr. said it was just a coincidence and that I needed to be careful because it could spike again. I continued to take coconut oil (organic type) for another 3 weeks. This time when I was tested my TSH was down to 4.2 . . . . My thyroid is back to normal and I lost all the weight I had gained and even gained muscle in the process, without even working out! Since then, I have continued to do research on the healing properties of coconut oil and can't stop talking to everyone about it."

—

I think that's pretty amazing! We now have and use organic virgin coconut oil for cooking, and I put it in my organic irish oats also, incorporating it as much as I could. Organic refined coconut oil has no coconut aroma, organic unrefined coconut oil has a coconutty one. I've used it for a butter substitute in solid form when baking, and melted as oil when needed. It does have multiple benefits and good effects, so I would encourage you to simply google "benefits of coconut oil" for yourself and you will be amazed as well I think.

April 2013

So What exactly is Hypothyroidism?

The thyroid gland is a butterfly-shaped gland in the front of the neck (right below the adams apple). Hypothyroidism is a condition in which the thyroid gland does not produce enough thyroid hormones. A healthy thyroid produces the hormones thyroxine (T4) and triiodothyronine (T3), which control metabolism. This affects how many calories you burn, how warm you feel, how much you weigh, and how the body handles functions of the cardiovascular, gastrointestinal, and nervous systems. Hypothyroidism results in a slower metabolism and a slower heartbeat.

And, What Causes Hypothyroidism?

I often hear regarding an illness or disease the details perhaps of what exactly happens in the body, but not so much on *what initally causes it? or why* one get's what they get? In which case I'd always scratch my head wondering. As I suspected earlier in my commentary what I personally believed, here is what researchers at the Centers for Disease Control and Prevention have found regarding hypothyroidism:

"American women, and *especially women with low iodine intake*, are at risk of hypothyroidism due to common exposure to the *toxin perchlorate*." Hmmmm

"Perchlorate is a byproduct of rocket fuel production and found to contaminate drinking water supply, as well as fruits, vegetables and grains irrigated by perchlorate-contaminated water, and milk and milk products from cows that grazed on contaminated grasses."

"Perchlorate can inhibit the thyroid's ability to absorb iodine from the bloodstream. Researchers found the presence of perchlorate was predictive of thyroid hormone levels in women—but not men. In women with higher-iodine levels, they found a slight connection between perchlorate levels and TSH (Thyroid Stimulating Hormone). But in the lower-iodine women, there was a strong connection between perchlorate levels, and elevated TSH and low T4—indicative of hypothyroidism.

—

Is that the reason for much of the weight problems today?

Interestingly my original commentary was written in March 2012 long before finding the above information in this case a study indeed showing specifically which chemical (percholorate) is in the environment and food supply itself, and one of the actual *culprits* that may be *causing* the serious weight and hormonal problems of *millions* of women and wanted to share it here as well. I *hope* this helps raise everyone's awareness of where at least some illness comes from again, (some form of toxicity or deficiency (or both) the importance of taking in less toxic foods, (going organic) and in hypothyroidism case, the thing that is being depleted is iodine, and is perhaps needed for your thyroid to function properly.

Patti aka: rustichealthy

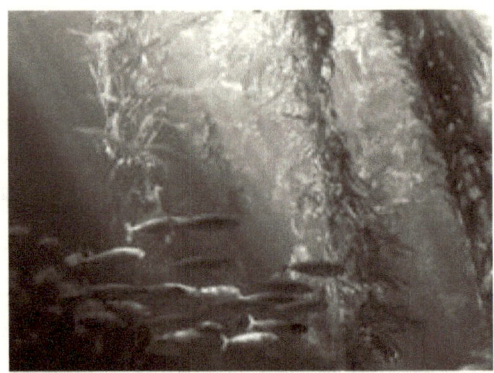

Kelp is a natural source of iodine and can be found in supplement form also. However, it is not the only cause. Always check with your medical doctor before taking iodine supplements to determine if iodine deficiency is related to your particular condition. If your doctor does recommend iodine supplementation, there are a few natural sources of iodine you can include in your diet. Both kelp and bladderwrack are sea plants rich in iodine.

Recommended Dietary Allowance for iodine is about 150 micrograms a day. The thyroid gland may try to procure iodine from the bloodstream which creates an enlarged thyroid gland, or goiter. On the other hand, too much iodine in the diet can cause an increased concentration of thyroid stimulating hormones in the body. The resulting condition is known as toxic goiter. Please check with your doctor on how much you should/shouldn't be taking also.

A few other vitamins and nutrients to look into for hypothyroid are:

Vitamin D3, (and get some *Sun*)!

B Vitamins are a group of eight nutrients responsible for cell metabolism. B complex vitamins can be taken as a daily supplement, or you can obtain them by consuming whole grains, dark green leafy vegetables, fish, poultry and other meat products. The University of Maryland Medical Center recommends avoiding certain foods that may actually interfere with thyroid function. These include foods such as broccoli, cabbage, cauliflower, kale, spinach, turnips, peanuts, linseed, pine nuts, millet and mustard greens. You should also avoid soy products as they are known to interfere with the absorption of thyroid hormones. Going into vegan forums, I also learned of Nutritional Yeast as another good source for B Vitamins.

Omega 3s (Flax oil is one source, and another good source is krill oil)

11 Foods that may help Speed your *Metabolism*

Hot Peppers
Broccoli
Green Tea
Spices
Foods High in Calcium
Purified Water

Whole Grains
Soups
Apples & Pears
Citrus Fruits
Foods High in Omega 3s

Rustic Commentary 2

The Newest "Scape Goat"

April 2012

I suppose everyone has heard (over and over and over *ad nauseum:*) that in the diet and food world that 'HFCS' (High Fructose Corn Syrup) is now the newest *'enemy' and 'culprit'* which I refer to as the "newest scapegoat" of health and weight loss! It started with calories, (there's a difference between good calories and bad calories). Then it was whole eggs, (however it's found the yoke is where the nutrients are, and it is not the cause of the bad cholesterol afterall). Then it went to fats, (but there are good fats that are very necessary like the omegas). Then it went to 'carbs', (but there are very good carbs necessary for your health). Then any and all red meat, (yet grass fed free range beef has nutrients you need, omegas and B vitamins, you can't find readily in a plant based diet) and now . . . it's high fructose corn syrup! HFCS is now your #1 enemy!

I shared from "Go Organic" and throughout the book how it wasn't until I cut out t o x i n s, and by going *organic,* that is when I actually returned to some 'normalcy' regarding food, weight loss and health. I had help for quite a while, with vitamins at the least, and I am most thankful for it! They held down my asthma and arthritis and some other things, but I never found a way to deal with my weight problem :/! Not until I went *organic,* and with even less 'exercise' :p then I've done prior to it! Actually, very little, although I do believe it's better to be active quickly I add!

The mayor of NYC is now proposing a 'ban' on large regular soda drinks. No . . . *not "diet"* drinks with all their *carcinogenic* chemicals in them :/ Hmmmm. Unfortunately, it is half right. *HFCS is* bad for you and for everyone as a matter of fact (not only those with weight problems)!.

It's one of the foods that are most likely gmo'd for one. It's the *t o x i n s* (pesticides, hormones, antibiotics, now gmos) in the production and growth of non-organic corn (where HFCS is from) in addition to most fruits, vegetables, chickens/cattle now fed with them. And, then there's all the artificial coloring, flavoring, preservatives of processed food and soda in the non-organic world that are the real enemy. Not the whole natural organic food itself! And it's not you! T o x i n s and chemicals never seem to be something made an issue in the multi stream media, or conventional researchers and/or health specialists. Well I'm making a big issue of it here! :) It's not sugar (HFCS), fats, carbs, beef and eggs! No, it's *what's being done to them* in it's process (added hormones, antibiotics, pesticides, etc.) that are the *real* culprit. So, what will the "food police" of the conventional medical and drug, food and diet world use as a "scapegoat" next? I wonder Hmmmm

"Scapegoat: *The secret of success is knowing who (and what) to blame*".

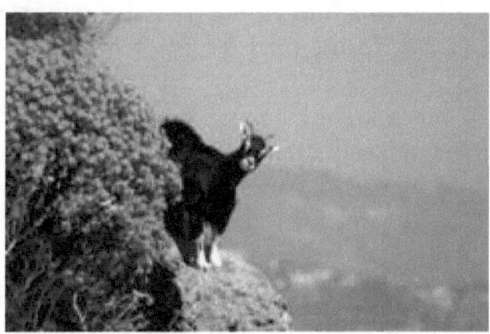

Rustic Commentary 3

Whose Guinea Pig are You?

May 2012

The fellow who has not had any experience is so dumb he doesn't know a thing can't be done, and he goes ahead and does it. (Well that fits me!:)

I've been away for a week, having moved recently and just getting back on line (which I missed dreadfully). I didn't move far, but funny it was practically as physical and stressful an ordeal as moving a few states! however, we did make it! I discovered not having any experience, that I can actually drive a 26 foot moving van too! :)

During the moving "ordeal", I was thinking of this, and I wanted to share it. In "About the Author" I stated, *"Basically, I've been my own guinea pig"*. What I don't think most realize is, we've actually all been unwittingly, unknowingly and *unfortunately 'guinea pigs' in the health fields* :(Considering all that I've shared here, especially in "What Do We Get?" and "Just Say No :/" we need to determine *whose* guinea pig we wish to be now regarding our *own* health. I know how much better I've been trying out wholefood supplements and vitamins in these years getting off of asthma and arthritis meds, and going organic, (as my son has now too), in essence being *my own* "guinea pig". I didn't *know* initially if Vitamin C would help. I didn't *know* if calcium would help me as it did the pain suffering woman I told. We didn't *know* if it would necessarily help my son either and his constant allergies and headaches as well. You have to simply be willing to try something 'unconventional' (yet safe please) for yourself.

So that's my thought, "We're all "guinea pigs", *whose* do you want to be?" I hope you don't let others experiment on you unknowingly, concerning your own health now anymore! Get different opinions. Do your *own* research. Don't be corraled or bullied into any already "acceptable" treatment. Look to see if there are other *safer, healthier* alternatives for everything, right down to a sniffle! One doctor online, wrote this: **"Ultimately, you must come to the realization that YOU are responsible for your, and your family's health—not me, not your physician, and certainly not any researchers or government health agencies that are beholden to the drug industry."** I couldn't agree more! And another put it this way: **"If you want something done right, you have to do it yourself. This especially includes your health care!"**. Why especially your healthcare? Because it's *you, it's your* life, and you are the one to have to live with it (and pay for it) for the rest *of your* life.

I recently found this comment regarding how another drug was now being put out without any testing . . .

"This is totally unacceptable. I have worked in the health care field for over 50 years, and back in the 1950's a drug was tested for 15+ years before put on the market. (I didn't know that) **As years passed the years shortened and now it is out of the factory today and tomorrow people are the "testors" not rats or guinea pigs** . . . . **We need to make a statement to congress,** . . . . **!!!!"**

:) Whether we write our congressmen or not, you can *still* choose who you personally listen to, and be sure of what goes in your *own* and your family's body, and health. My conclusion here is, in the conventional food and health world, "We are *all* 'guinea pigs', so whose do you want to be?" . . .

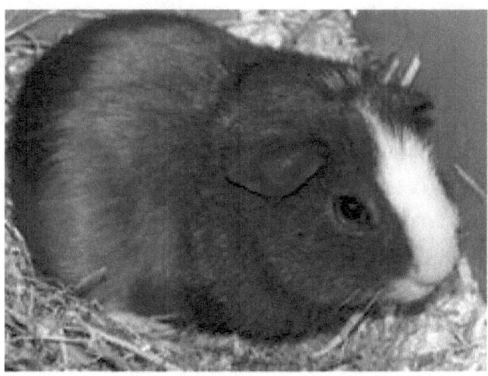

Patti aka: rustichealthy being my own *healthy* . . . :)

Rustic Commentary 4

Bad Medicine:/ in the "Belly of the Beast" and the "Dose of the Vitamin"

May 2012

I've been in a debate (attack & defense:) recently on another conventional med site I now refer to as "The Belly of the Beast":) It is a forum hosted by a few conventional doctors. Both doctors and medical students (for the most part it seems) are found there, a few nurses perhaps, some other professionals, and now . . . there was me! :) I had gone over because I heard of *their "concern and outrage"* of a woman and how she was considering choosing to go with an alternative doctor and remedy, to help with her very aggressive stage 3 breast cancer. And interestingly the husband himself was there also, whom they were "debating" some berating him! :/ . . . and so this is where I entered . . .

"I guess the rage in the OP is what I find interesting. The patient had already undergone treatment, that had not worked, actually gotten worse, and you're outraged that she would consider another way? Or, . . . you're outraged that she has the opportunity to use other methods, and that others have different views and answers to cancer . . . . The prospects of her new treatment, the doctors recommended were not good. Maybe . . . a few months? and have to go through what they proposed? . . . . and I quoted what the woman stated were all the astounding horrific effects, and side-effects of chemo and radiation treatment . . ." . . . . **treatments may or may not cure this, they may only extend my life by a few months, the cancer may return, I would most likely suffer heart damage, the irreversible**

106

shut down of my hormones, the destruction of my immune system, the loss of my lymph nodes, my energy, my breasts (would likely remove the other as precautionary), my hair temporarily, and the list went on and on . . . I would head into surgery with no immune system and then when I'd recovered from that blow to my body, I would undergo rounds and rounds of radiation, and while healing from the trauma of that I would be put back on chemo therapy and my immune system again would be destroyed, and if I ever got sick while on these treatments it would be a life or death emergency." . . . and . . .

"What the doctors were CERTAIN about were the side effects. In fact, we heard about 3 hours worth of side-effects related to their proposed treatments. They said, "so, the cancer may grow resistant to the treatments we bombard it with. We can pretty much guarantee heart damage, with a side of intestinal destruction, and we know we can absolutely destroy your immune system and anything else your body could use to heal. And to top it off, you get to lose your hair, have no energy and walk around like a zombie". and I continued . . .

Why the Op is not *outraged* at those things is what I don't know. :) anyway . . . my personal belief is . . . cancer is a response to toxins . . . things that do not belong in our bodies to begin with. My site has a lot on it so, I'm asking the OP (not certain if you are a doctor or not) if you would like to please visit it. It has my own experience, that does not "comply" to conventional medicine as well . . . sorry :) I got off of 4 asthma meds because of my 'unconventional' experiments . . . i.e. started taking vitamins instead . . . as well as other things . . . . and, without the use of the internet at the time." . . . .

And so I entered *"the Belly of the Beast"* . . . of course the conventional medical doctors and students there were questioning my *own* experience, dismissing everything I say as "anecdotal" and/or "placebo", along with any other alternative remedies I tried to offer. The conventionals there felt and also claimed there was (or should be) *no decision* to be made by the husband and wife! . . . actually it was *their* way or the highway! . . . *(that* disturbed me). The 'discussion' went on for days afterward! I then this morning opened an email regarding the huge amount of deaths (over a 100,000 a year?) from conventional medications themselves taken *as prescribed* . . .

Medical care is actually one of the leading causes of death in the U.S., with medical errors, adverse drug reactions, and hospital-acquired infections killing an unacceptable number of

Americans each and every day. Drug-related ER visits jumped by more than half between 2004 and 2008 stirring health officials to look for ways to stop what has *become a near-epidemic that often ends in death.*

. . . . I did try sharing how one was healed with a simple mixture of baking soda, molasses and water! (Always a mistake to bring up in a conventional medical forum by the way:) Of course that was dismissed easily. However, if you see the video on youtube for yourself, and go to Vern's website, phkillscancer.com I think you will find it believable, but you should decide for *yourself!* I fail to see the reason for this man with stage 4 prostate cancer, or any of the other people I've read about online, share their own testimony freely. What would be the purpose? You might say one or two are trying to get publicity from it, or mistaken, or delusional, etc., but 100's? 1000's? of testimonies and freely given information of all different simple remedies and experiences? I think the more you hear the better, and it's up to you whether to look into something or not, before dismissing them for *yourself* (and not someone else making that decision *for* you). Remember, it's *your* health, not anyone elses! The husband of the woman above happened to come into the forum himself trying to show how *they* were the ones to decide what was right for them and what wasn't! That they (those on the forum) were jumping to conclusions. But, the conventionals there were *appalled* that *anything else* would even be *considered.* The harsh comments, and coming from those who purported to somehow believe they actually knew and cared more for his wife then he did! (consider the side-effects stated) It was surreal to say the least.

I do not know all of what the apparently alternative doctor prescribes for the above, I was mostly trying to address the outrage over anyone going to alternative treatment, instead of taking conventional medical advice *only*, (in this case concerning chemo and radiation, the standard go-to treatment for most any inoperable cancer), of probably living like a zombie for 3 more months *IF* she survives their bombardment on her body with conventional chemo and radiation 'treatments', while calling all alternatives "dangerous" and "evil"?! Based on the medical errors, adverse drug reactions, and hospital-acquired infections actually *killing* an unacceptable number of Americans each and every day, why do conventional medicals feel so superior to any alternative treatment I wonder. The usual defense is well, "It's the *dose* of the poison" prescribed, and their "risk vs. benefit" ratio . . . (or their *idea* of it anyway) and we're supposed to simply 'trust' their judgement on that still, without question, o boy.

"It's the Dose of the Vitamin" then!

While conventional medicals usually claim *"It's the Dose of the Poison"* that matters in their prescription of chemical medicines inevitably in conversation, one will point out the danger of *vitamins*. When I shared how calcium with Vit. D and magnesium have been *helping me* for years, (rather than pain meds) for arthritis, one pointed out, "calcium can affect your heart, calcitrate your arteries". Which troubled me a little. It turns out in the study they were referring to, calcium supplements were given mostly to women who smoked . . . Hmmm There are many other variables to take into consideration (remember to take calcium supplements *with* magnesium to help it absorb better) I believe that are not possible to show (possibly omitted) in every test all the time and I no longer am concerned with conventional studies to prove or disprove anything now.

Orthomolecular Medicine News Service, January 5, 2011

***Zero Deaths* from Vitamins, Minerals, Amino Acids or Herbs: Poison Control Statistics Prove Supplements' Safety Yet Again**
(OMNS Jan 5, 2011) There was *not even one death* caused by a dietary supplement in 2009, according to the most recent information collected by the U.S. National Poison Data System.

—

Now when a conventional tries to alarm me with how vitamins are *"dangerous"*, my answer to them will be well, *"It's the Dose of the Vitamin"* *then!* And it's my own "risk/benefit ratio". Doesn't that dismiss everything else?

Please note also, *low* Vitamin D levels have been linked with breast cancer. The *lower* the Vitamin D, the more *aggressive the cancer.* Supplementing with Vitamin D is *very* important especially during winter months, and being out of the sun. Vitamin D3 is the natural source. The sun itself of course is the *best source*! I'm using also a calcium with magnesium and Vitamin D supplement as well.

So, my message here is, it's you foremost to decide what route you wish to go in your own health and please don't be intimidated, coralled or bullied otherwise!

rustichealthy from inside . . . *"the Belly of the Beast"* :)

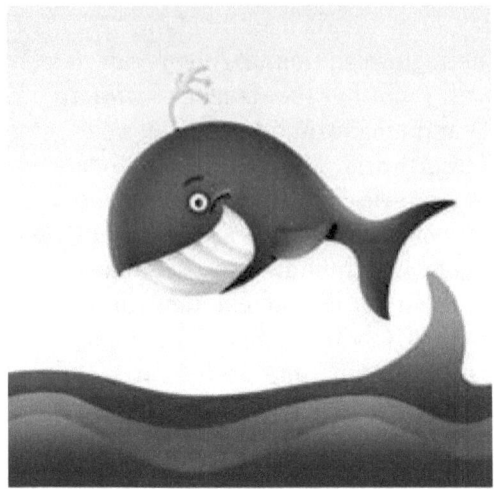

"If we doctors threw all our medicines into the sea, it would be that much better for our patients and that much worse for the fishes." Oliver Wendell Holmes, M.D.

Rustic Commentary 5

"Liar, Fraud!"

June 2012

"Liar, Fraud"! (?) Yes, that's what I've been called in the conventional world of "health & healing" just from going organic, taking vitamins and wanting *and/or trying* to help others in this area. In particular when I relay what happened to me in the only one 'cold incident' I've had now in over four years now (thankfully). In "It's A LivingStyle" I spoke of the small lump that somehow 'disappeared' 6 months later also. I did say keep in mind I had for a long while been taking vitamins every day (doubled in that time). In my 1 Hour Cold incident (on "It's Take Time") I had been about 80% organic diet (which I believe helps) at that time, and taking vitamins and nutrients every day as well, building up my immune system "muscles" so at the time when I needed a little *extra* reinforcements . . . they worked! A weight lifter doesn't pick up 200 lbs in just one day of 'training' and muscle building, no, it takes time to build up to it. They weren't just some unique magical instances of amazing strength or fluke, which then seem to result in accusations of "liar, fraud" from some conventionals anyway.

Clinical trials that are taken, of what vitamins work, or how well they work are really difficult to satisfy the 'science-based' thinking conventional medical doctors and students. "Insufficient or Inconclusive Evidence" is the usual conclusion. They may have tested let's say 200 mg. of Vit. C (in ascorbic acid) (I take 1000 a day minimum with bioflavanoids and rosehips) so, what would their tests show to me? of course 200 mg of Vit. C (in ascorbic acid) may not be effective on me. We're all amazingly different. It's not really possible to say in my opinion what or how much works for one, works for another. I may get an idea what to use, and go with it (as

I did with Vit. C for asthma). For me, 2 or 3 1000 mgs per day may have been needed some days at the time, for another only 500 mg a day. There can be no real specifics in my thinking, since everyone is in a different health condition, a different diet, at a different age, a different environment, even a different day . . . or season! It's a matter of simply building your own immune system 'muscles' the best you can on a daily basis, (like the weight lifter) to the amount you need for yourself and *your* environment, and to be ready for any 'outside attacks' when they come and may have to increase them perhaps? Unfortunately, you will be called a "Liar and a Fraud" too if and when you share of your own successful experience most likely, just as they do with any personal experience of mine or others I've shared and heard. Totally dismissed by conventionals as simply "anecdotal" or "placebo" most times.

Everyone outside of conventional "chemical based medicine" is a "quack" in their minds it seems anyway. It's too bad *how closed minded* they've become in their 'science' based medicine. There's 'good' science, and there's 'bad' science in my mind. The difference is, alternatives use more *'do no harm'* methods and substances most times. However, a few things came up lately, and so I would implore anyone and everyone to really look into something first, yes even in the alternative world, before trusting yourself into the hands of others (even alternatives) without question, or even myself and what I say! I saw on "Myth Busters" just yesterday 'testing' if they could swallow a heaping tablespoon of cinnamon with nothing to drink. With or *without* something to drink it is *not* something you do! without other information and counsel! Still, considering the track record and adverse effects of regular prescription drugs "taken as prescribed" in my previous post, it's very odd to hear conventional medicals bring up the *'danger'* of vitamins and alternatives! Anyway, that's my rambling for today. Just be ready for the "liar and fraud" accusations slung at you too! *Go Organic, take your vitamins,* and still be happy getting healthy!:)

Patti aka: rustichealthy Liar, Fraud

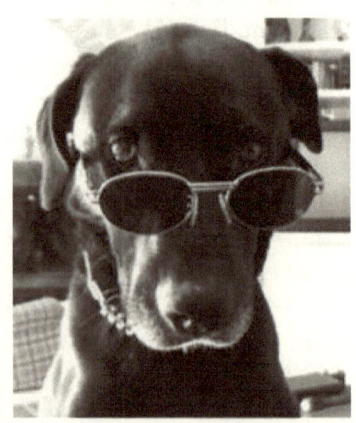

Please remember: Vitamin supplements may have allergy affects in rare cases. Some vitamin supplements may also conflict with any medications you are taking as well. Always consult with your doctor before taking them.

One of my answers to this question and some other comments in the *"Belly of the Beast"* . . .

"How about it Rustic? What would you consider to be sufficient to get you to change your mind about what you have been discussing? Purely hypothetically speaking of course—what can you possibly imagine could be presented to you that would make you realize and admit you are wrong?"

That's a curious question to me. How can I admit I'm "wrong" about my own experience(?) . . . how do I answer that . . ."Yes I am wrong . . . , I took vitamin C and it worked, but I admit I am wrong that it worked" (?) or for saying "it worked"(?) this is what I answered . . . .

. . .

This is the thing . . . if someone gives their experience . . . isn't it "polite" :) to at least say . . . "hmmm . . . I don't know about that" . . . "we'll have to look into it". What if your patient said that . . . "doctor . . . this and this happened". Would you ask him for a "clinical study"? on it first before believing him? tell him he's a "moron, idiot, it's not in my books . . . etc etc. . . ."? That's what I had to think about when I went to the doctors . . . not to tell them what happened and how I'm feeling better. It's strange to me to hear from those who are into 'healing' be so closed and ornery sometimes, when something is against what they are taught 'healing' is . . . which in con(ventional) meds case is what the pharmas say it seems. I'd understand if you all had stock in pharmas . . . ok then . . . I'd get it.:) But, I don't believe that's the case either for most.

Where's the 'science' in denying so many many things . . . honestly . . . 1000's having other home remedies that worked, because their doctor's medicine didn't . . . . please . . . go to EarthClinic.com and tell me that all those people are "lunatics, morons, *liars*, *frauds*, idiots" etc . . . when they speak of their own

natural remedies they've tried and worked . . . (one taking olive oil and lemon juice to relieve painful kidney stones that they had no relief from in medicines) on illnesses that only seem to get worse in con med world . . . like hbp, diabetes, even cancer . . . when nothing else did. Can you all honestly say "well . . . it's just not clinically tested! so therefore it isn't?"

I don't have all the tests, information, labs, etc. to prove anything I say. I'm only amazed at the reactions and accusations and allegations I've gotten since going on line and speaking of them. Now I'm accused of actually being "*dangerous*"?! wow . . . considering how I then read how *Millions* are dead because of "taking their prescriptions . . . as prescribed" . . . and I'm "*dangerous*"(?)

Just to be clear . . . I didn't say Vit. C was the *only* vitamin I took . . . *it was the first*, and it did help . . . but not entirely . . . I had to find others. There were no books or other information I had. I'm not saying it works for all, I'm saying it's *something to look into*, and maybe there are other things that would help, things that are less *truly* dangerous than substances like steroids and antibiotics, etc. It's too bad, but, most people are left to find out for *themselves*, and not from their doctors.

—

Another question:
"**Forgive us Rusty, we're honestly confused about what you mean by "toxin". I take it vitamins, like the one that cured your asthma, is not a toxin . . . right?**"
Was that a trick question? hmmmm . . . After being told (*quite a few times*) that "vitamins and nutrients" *were just as much* "toxins" as conventional medicines are . . . I gave up . . .
**. . . "if I said it was a "*toxin*" . . . would you all then be okay with it"(?) would it then be an acceptable remedy (?) "Yes okay! . . . Vitamin C is a *"Toxin"*! . . . I'm not sure what it is still with *"toxins"* and conventional medicals! :)

Rustic Commentary 6

Why Do My Placebos Work?

June 2012

Many times I've been also informed by conventionals that vitamins, nutrients, and probably everything else I've done (and what others I've known did), are all "placebos". I give an example of my own experience? . . . "Placebo!" Of someone else's experience? . . . "Placebo!" Of 1000s of other's experiences? . . . "Placebos"! We're all "Delusionary, Uneducated, and Brainwashed". Actually, I read in one of the blogs that they're considering that we (those that claim their alternatives just so happened to work, and where illness just so 'happened to go away') have a special kind of "placebo gene"(?) Well, I would like to address this here and now! It's taken long and difficult, disciplined and laborious years to perfect my health and healing *skill*. And so if my vitamin C didn't help with my asthma and colds at the time I needed them? Then I *willed* them to work, and, so . . . they did! If my calcium supplements didn't help with mine (or my friend's mother-in-law's) arthritis, (or my heartburn when I took it)? Then I *willed* them to work, and so . . . they did! If changing to organic foods didn't address the insane battle I had with food for all these years, or allergies, or asthma, I simply *willed* it to work and so . . . it did! *And* it 'worked' for my son's allergies and headaches too! And for the woman who took my 'suggestion' of calcium for her arthritis? and for another with apple cider vinegar and hemorrhoids? and another with Vit C and her asthma? . . . Well, I am really darned good at this! I happened to be watching a little of a rerun of Star Wars the other day, and . . . That's it! I have my answer . . . It is a sign! Why do *my 'placebos'* work? becuz, . . . *Ssstrong* am I in the *'Placebo' force!* :)) heh

Patti: aka rusticjedi :)

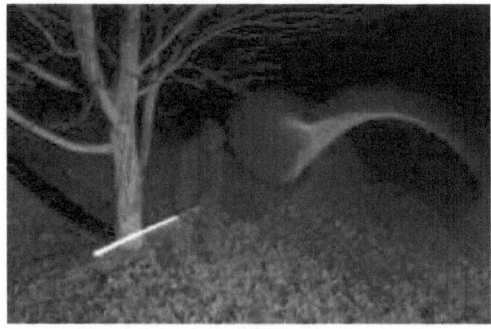

"May the *"placebo force"* be with you also!" :)

===

Rustic Commentary 7

Vegan/Vegetarian or Organic Omnivore

June 2012

While I do agree (naturally) that eating healthy fresh foods, vegetables and dairy (for vegetarians) are better than a normal processed food diet (more fresh fruits/vegetables and hopefully less processed foods with preservatives and artificial ingredients) it seems to be rarely spoken of, or made a point in any case, of *"organic"* fruits/vegetables and dairy among vegans and vegetarians. Vegans and vegetarians who do so because they're protesting any killing of animals for food, or in their belief man is not meant to be omnivorous (I would disagree) but then ok fine, that is their belief . . . I just want to say maybe consider 'organic' also, fruits/vegetables and dairy, with less pesticides, hormones, etc. that do kill the environment (and other animals and insects) actually, and still more healthy for you! If it's solely for 'health' then I'd wonder why not consider *"organic"* and make it a point also? I'm neither vegan nor vegetarian though I have more of a "plant based diet" now because organic meats and poultry are not readily available in the market near me, (I have found *wild caught* (not farm raised) fish and shrimp however in the fish/frozen section) and it is pretty expensive for me to order all the time. I do support more *humane treatment* of all animals of course like free range chickens and cattle and against CAFOs. I'd argue if *it's only* because you believe killing is "inhumane practice" to consider all of nature is "inhumane" then? animals killing other animals for food also. In any case we all have and should continue to have the right and freedom to choose what we want going in our bodies and not to legislate or mandate others to do what we believe is so, always, in a free country and society that is. My *cause* would be to have a more *healthy non-toxic* food supply for *all*, vegan, vegetarian and omnivore. What is being forced on us all now unawares for the most part is chemical laden, genetically modified lab created foods, pesticides, hormones and antibiotic laden non-organic food to begin with. I believe we should and could all "join forces" and rally for *healthy non-toxic food*, fruit, vegetable or meat and dairy, whatever diet we choose!

Patti aka: rusticomnivore

The "Circle of Life" or "Night of Terror in the Country"

While living at a ranch several years ago, I was awoken at around 2 a.m. The terrorized wild screeching of one of the free range roosters, who used to walk freely among the grass with his friends, pecking and picking up bugs and worms swallowing them whole. Living and working in NYC, we were used to the screeching of sirens and the screeching of subway trains, but not this. No, not this. It was a happy life (pity the bugs and worms who had a life of their own albeit). He usually flew up in the trees at night like his friends as well, but, didn't do so for some reason on this awful, awful "night of terror in the country", and no one knows why. A fox now had him in his jaws, carrying him around and around the house, screeching and fluttering, over and over and over, until the poor rooster gave in and finally died, in the jaws of the fox, (ending up being a tasty meal for the fox). It was a terrifying incident, but, everything naturally and ecologically, is for a reason and necessity, and everything unfortunately dies at some point in time, whether it end up on a dinner plate, or in the jaws of a predator. No, it is not always "humane". No it is not always without suffering and loss, but it is the means of sustenance and survival. It is . . . *the "Circle of Life."* I would choose to have humane treatment of *all* animals, ending quick and painless as possible, having them lived a happy and decent free life as much as possible too. A free range organic happy life. I believe we can all agree on that. :)

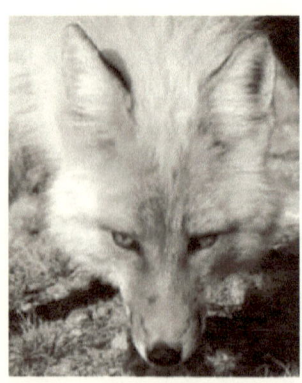

One of Aesop's Fables of Foxy Rooster

A fox sneaked into a farm and grabbed a prize rooster.

The farmer saw him and raised the alarm and he and his dogs started chasing the thief.

The fox, though he was holding the rooster in his mouth, was running very fast.

"Get him! Get him!" shouted the farmer to his dogs.

"No!" suddenly screamed the rooster. "Don't come near me!"

"My master was very cruel to me," explained the rooster to the fox. "Tell him to stay away from me."

The fox was delighted. "He wants you to stay away from him!" he shouted at the farmer, in the process releasing his hold on the rooster.

The rooster flew up into a tree and stayed there till he was rescued by his master.

Moral: Think twice before you open your mouth to speak.

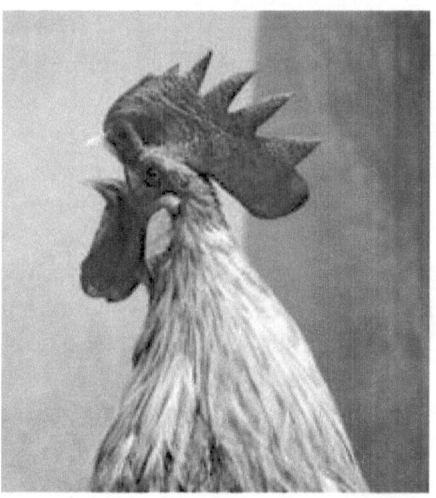

I actually put the above 2 "stories" in the vegan forum now called "Veganville" to answer one's theory that all carnivores (and omnivores) would die out . . . well . . . there's more on that in "Defending Omnivores . . . Taking on the Vegans":)

Rustic Commentary 8

What's the Harm Rethink

June 1012

Now, to be "fair and balanced", I was referred to a site called "What's the Harm", by a conventional m.d. in "the Belly of the Beast" (the aforementioned conventional medical forum). I did go and I did find things that I believe everyone should be aware of and consider when doing anything regarding home remedies and alternatives (as well as conventional by the way). Be aware of the harms done by conventional *and* alternatives as well. I've said things like "No one should swallow a heaping tablespoon of cinnamon". It is a powerful natural antibiotic but that doesn't mean *it's harmless* if taken too much of at once, or incorrectly. ("it's the dose of the vitamin?") At the time a man was challenged to take a heaping tablespoon of cinnamon on a late night show. He did, and was successfully happy doing so, and everyone clapped and cheered. But when he was sitting back down in the audience, I kept looking, and you can see a strange look on his face, in his eyes, that he did not feel well at all. So my point here is, if you are looking into a specific alternative, consult your doctor or health professional first, and you can as well look up "What's the Harm" on the internet, and peruse the site to see what may be some things to look for that could be detrimental even natural vitamins and nutrients (like cinnamon) if taken too much of perhaps. There is an old saying "Don't put all your eggs in one basket". That's exactly what I would do also with alternatives, vitamins, etc. Find out the down sides as well. I would not put all my hope in one nutrient, herb remedy or vitamin, either. I did in the beginning relying mostly on Vitamin C but, I found out for myself I needed others also! Actually, as you know probably by now:) I believe we need all vitamins and nutrients, and preferably in their closest natural state in whole foods or whole food supplements (and preferably organic).

So, as always, look over, study, get other professional advice and counsel if needed. Don't jump into something unknown without *careful* study, even things like bee pollen (some may very well have a bad allergic reaction), colloidal silver (some have actually *turned* silver). Go slow to be sure of anything that you are not familiar with personally. I have gotten tired of conventional medicals warnings about anything alternative, that I've been very defensive about *all alternatives*, because of the attacks and trying to stop and silence everyone who is into them! But I want to make it clear that that doesn't mean *all* alternatives are harmless! Personally I would get properly diagnosed by a conventional doctor, get a second opinion if I needed to, understand my choices, and seek out as best I could a natural and organic wholefood or other natural remedy also. I personally like EarthClinic.com, to see all the different real and personal "anecdotal" experiences, (from those who are not getting paid for it), and no other motive than to share what they've experienced! I don't see *any* harm in *going all organic* though, only good! So, keep it safe, keep it balanced, and keep informed for yourself of the downsides of both alternative and conventional.

Patti aka: rusticrethinking :)

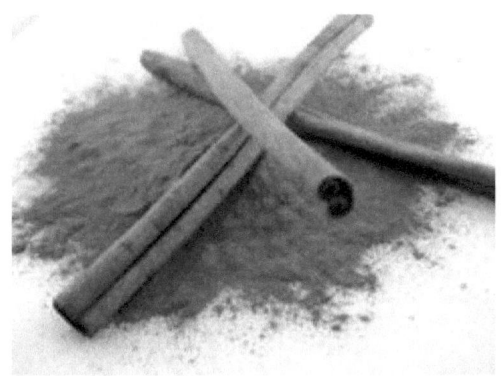

Some great health benefits of cinnamon?

Balances Blood Sugar
Promotes Weight Loss
Helps Your Heart
Fights Cognitive Decline
Keeps Cells Healthy
Soothes Inflammation
Fights Infections

Please Note: Vitamin supplements may have allergy affects in rare cases (even cinnamon). Some vitamin supplements may also conflict with any medications you are taking as well. Always check with your doctor before taking cinnamon or any other vitamin and nutrient.

==

Rustic Commentary 9

The Belly of the Beast and "Green Coffee Beans"

July 2012

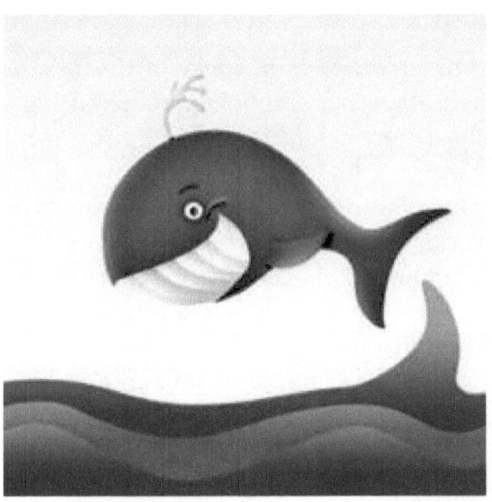

"It's a strangely stupid new world we are coming into." That's my conclusion after another few days in the "Belly of the Beast", this time the topic was weight loss and organic foods. Actually, it started on the topic "Dr. Oz and Green Coffee Beans". Dr. Oz had recently aired a program on it. Most of their comments were criticizing and mocking the "green coffee bean" claims. So, of course, I had to then put in my *own* two beans:) and

told how I was *not* defending green coffee beans for weight loss, but that *going organic* was the way I was able to begin losing weight anyway. It started out friendly enough! Someone (new to me there) even wanting to have a 'clinical trial' to see if organic foods would have an effect as I was claiming it did (for myself anyway). I gave a site where it gives all the chemicals, hormones and antibiotics that are in our regular foods and how they may affect many people.

However, *being in the "Belly of the Beast" as it were*, it then quickly *"descended to the depths"* from there! Now I have no delusions of my own intellect, and I heavens do not dispute that these people are much more *educated* than I am anyway :) but, seriously? What I heard once again were some of the most ridiculous to the absurd! Some were the usual *"placebo"* (of course:) I'm still an *idiot* for not knowing that EVERYTHING is a chemical and/or toxin! (including organic foods and vitamins (?) and so there's therefore no difference between them and *other* toxic chemicals(?) :::sigh::: Did you know that? No difference! Then it was "Hey, there's toxins on your computer top!" (so therefore I shouldn't mind toxins in my food too(?)! I see :/ or "Gee, you can't make *your own* soap without lye yet?"(?) by one there who did this apparently, and therefore being so *incompetent*! and since I haven'*t cracked open a book* to find out how, I therefore should have nothing to say about toxins in my food and meds or body either! See? Okaay :/ . . .

One other (new to me there) then spoke of the 'new evolution' regarding GMOs when I brought them up, and how perhaps this is all part of it. We're "evolving" now into a new scientific evolution of 'synthetic' food supply and, how we could and should 'adapt' to the 'new evolution'! So, this is what the gmo and genically engineered mad scientists are trying to put it off as in the conventional world, because it certainly succeeded in the conventional 'belly of the beast' crowd! This new belief that we are *progressing*, that this is all part of the "new evolution", synthetic meds and synthetic foods, and those of us in the organic (real) food crowd are simply *archaic* and down right *primitive* cave men and women and *holding up progress* is what they seemed to be implying. Here's one regular there to my following statement . . .

"(I) . . . **refuse to see how organic natural foods have the same toxicity and chemicals as other toxic/chemical/man-made substances. I'm not sure how difficult that is to see . . . it's amusing to me frankly. Maybe that's my "organic" nature coming out :)"** . . .

"**No, it's not your "organic nature." It's because you are a blithering idiot. You have below average intelligence, likely bordering on handicapped. You are a fool.**" . . . :/ and then . . .

"I would be perfectly fine with someone removing rustic's ovaries so that she doesn't pass down whatever "dumb gene" she inherited. I mean, this is stupid to epic proportions."

Okay . . . that's it . . . and this is where I lost it :/ . . . after repeatedly trying to explain and refute 'civilly' as I could . . .

((***** (who is a doctor btw :) **"is the typical "smug, arrogant, condescending, judgemental" chemically filled conmed** (I call them) . . . **who apparently needs more chemical pills for psychotic reasons.**

I simply threw in my experience since green coffee beans and weight problems was the topic. I didn't expect the total attack on organic food too in here! I actually thought we could agree on *something* **. . . atleast in our food supply. I thought it perhaps contained itself to chemical meds. Now I know the goal is to have a total 'synthetic' (chemically toxic) foods . . . yes . . . I kind of suspected that., I just didn't think too many people would actually** *defend* **it, (!) but that's what I see in here too. Strangely stupid new world we are coming to."))**

Sorry, but what is really disturbing to me is the defense of it, even in "the belly of the beast"! They absolutely cannot bring themselves to say, "Hey, maybe a little *LESS* toxins wouldn't hurt us??" I honestly thought if they knew what was going in and on food (like gmos) they'd (being so much more intelligent and educated) at least want to consider a *little less* chemicals in their food supply too? right? No! Instead, they consider me ignorant and simply not "getting with the program", for **not** wanting them, and they defend e v e r y molecule of toxic poison they can! And, since I can't make my own soap (?) or know the name of all the chemicals and toxins in tobacco smoke (?) or I'm still sitting on a computer with "toxic dust", I therefore should be duct taped, drawn and quartered for rejecting them! I can't say how dumbfounded I am at this point :/. Anyway . . . that's all for now, from this last excursion . . .

Patti aka: rusticwearied

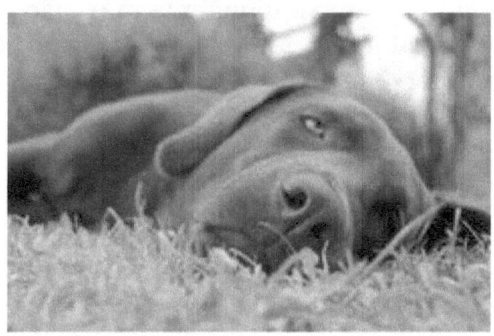

from . . . inside the "Belly of the Beast" :/ and

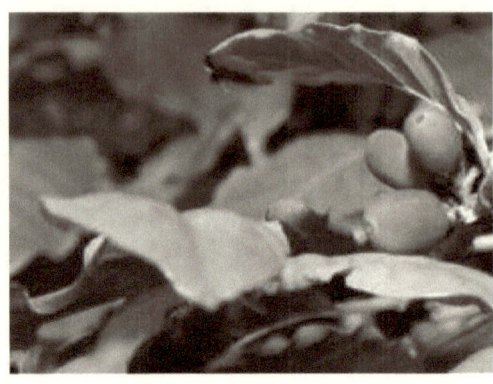

"Green Coffee Beans" :)

I did manage to have some energy to look up benefits reported of Green Coffee Beans though!

> High in Antioxidants
> Metabolism booster
> Burning of stored fat
> Lowering of blood pressure and cholesterol
> Powerful appetite suppressant
> Improved heart health
> Improved mental alertness
> Detoxifying liver
> Enhancing energy levels

> I may try them now afterall! :)

Please remember: Vitamin supplements may have allergy affects in rare cases. Some vitamin supplements may also conflict with any medications you are taking as well. Always consult with your doctor before taking them.

===

Rustic Commentary 10

Pain (Headache and Heartburn) Management

July 2012

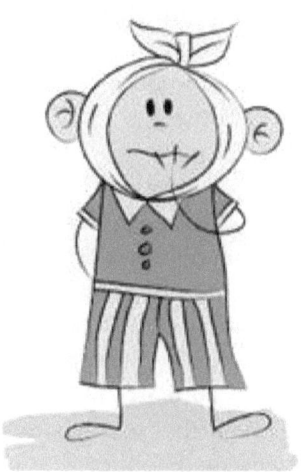

Recovering from my *last excursion* in 'the Belly of the Beast' :/ conventional medical forum, it is amazing that I didn't have a 'headache' (if I got them) for days afterwards:) Anyway, as I've mentioned, how I have a low tolerance to pain so I really do feel for anyone who's in much chronic pain. I personally can't imagine handling it for too long. I've found some articles on pain, on Rustic Healthy's home page "What's New" board and how to deal with it naturally, but I just wanted to add the following. Pain is an indication of something wrong (you may say obviously). But, it's something it seems to me, today, as I did myself all these years think and accept it as "normal" when you have even a slight headache? take some aspirin, heartburn? take an "antacid". However, I no longer believe it's something *normal or insignificant anymore*, not even something as a mild headache (though not always something serious). It is caused by something not right within the body! I saw on Dr. Oz how some headaches are from raised blood pressure to the brain, and so having something that lowers your blood pressure instead (such as some of the natural foods I have listed below) may be the thing to look into. Or some of the personal 'testimonies' I put below also. Personally I believe it may also have to do with yep, *toxins*, and yes in *non-organic* foods. Just an example . . .

For years I suffered from heartburn. Now I understand that would not be considered as "pain", but it's the only one I have actually that I personally can relate to. It actually felt sometimes like something was "cooking" in my throat on a regular basis, atleast two or three times a week. A 'burning' in my throat and chest area after eating certain foods though I never payed attention to exactly what they were. So you may say "Well, that would be the reason!" but there's a little more. As I've said before this, I would take a calcium supplement when I did and it would usually subside within a few minutes . . . it was great! Just one thing, now that I've gone mostly organic wholefood (about 80% now) I haven't had heartburn . . . at all! (ok except on an occasion when I ate too much non-organic food that is, at the holiday time; and yes, one time a few months ago I had a sleeve of non-organic oreo cookies:) :/ . . . lesson learned I think :)

Another is, my son used to get headaches pretty regularly, atleast every few weeks or so. I used to worry a bit as he wasn't really a 'complainer' (like myself it would be the hand to head (or head to table:) grief when I did have a rare headache) and he would barely mention them, but every once in a while he would have to lay down and rest because of it, fall asleep and it would go. I asked him a few weeks ago about his headaches and, nope! he has not had one in a long while! He can't remember actually, maybe 5 or 6 months . . . so he was happy about that too, besides the relief he's had about his allergies (without taking any meds either).

So my point here is, try to find out (if you don't know already) what it may be from (hint: possibly from non-organic foods?) as well as trying to deal with the pain (with a natural remedy) so that it won't come back and you'll be dealing with it from the source! Anyway, I hope this helps give a little more insight on it. It's not a lot, I don't have a lot, I'm a 'blithering idiot' afterall! but I hope it helps you think on a different level regarding pain i.e. headache and heartburn, and yes, arthritis, fibromyalgia (check out some testimonials on this) for a few others anyway. And to look for and find a more natural way of dealing with it for one, or perhaps even *eliminating* it by adding nutrients you may be lacking, changing your diet, or by simply going *organic*! (eliminating toxins) and then naturally preventing the cause to begin with! That would be my wish for you in order to be happy and to *healthily* fly high above any pain too . . .

Patti aka: rusticflying:) above pain *naturally*

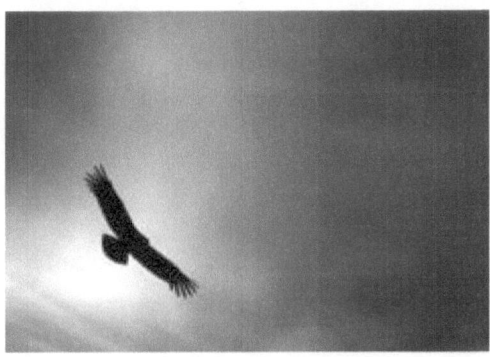

This is one who spoke of their terrible fibromyalgia pain, and what happened by simply going organic whole food!:

"digestion . . .

You can't feel good on all that medication. I've been suffering for years with digestive issues and fibromyalgia. So much so I went back to school at The Institute for Integrative Nutrition and became a health counselor.

After a great summer i started having more and more sensitivities to foods. And I'm not talking about processed foods. I'm talking about real whole home cooked foods. Everything seemed to bother me. I am now listening to what MY body needs which is a very simple easy to digest whole organic foods so that my body has time to heal and adjust to my age and lifestyle. Healing is a journey, a lifestyle into healthier living.

Coming off of the medication is only the beginning."

—

This is interesting, someone spoke of how his arthritis/fibromyalgia has been helped by taking a simple thing like cinnamon . . .

"Arthritis relief too simple to believe.

Wouldn't have tried this unless I'd seen it print. Cinnamon . . . that's all. My arthritis/fibromyalgia/RSD, whatever you want to call it, means I move around like a crab for a couple of hrs in the am, but taking 3 1000mg caps (available @ Sam's, or make your own) eliminates 80%+ of this most of the time.

Should have mentioned . . . . I take it @ bed time."

—

10 Healthy Things That can Lower Blood Pressure Today (and get rid of that mild headache naturally perhaps) organic as much as possible :)

Beets

Purple Potatoes

Black Tea

Chocolate

Squeezing a Rubber Ball

Grapes

Raisins

Vit. C

Soy

Exercise

Please remember: Vitamin supplements may have allergy affects in rare cases. Some vitamin supplements may also conflict with any medications you are taking as well. Always consult with your doctor before taking them.

_____
==

Rustic Commentary 11

Anecdotal vs. Clinical

July 2012

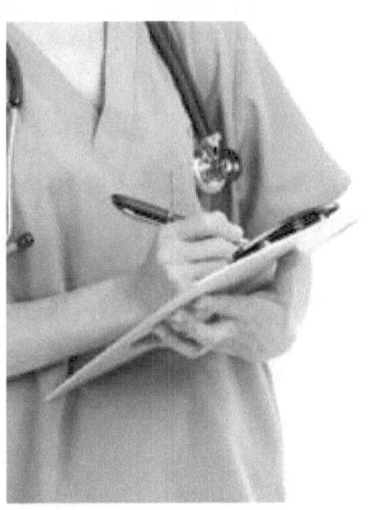

I've on many occasions tried sharing my personal experience with others online, only to be dismissed with "anecdotal" meaning it's simply my word and experience and nothing more. "Unscientific, unimportant, and meaningless", is what some were saying :/ Ok fine, so I'd try to find clinical trials on pubmed for one with 'conclusive evidence' to support my experience and actually rarely would find one, not in the conventional health world anyway, that would be accepted (although I find many others online that alternatives do conduct and accept). In my quest the other day on pubmed I came across one that said Vit. C (in ascorbic acid which is the one usually tested) had no effect on the regular population, . . . however! . . . in this one, it did have a *positive* effect on those in 'extreme' conditions, such as military, athletes, and the like. Aha . . . What was that? hmmmm. So, I wondered about this. What am I missing here? I thought this over a few minutes, talked this out with my son (the new organic health nut) as well and it came to us. Athletes and military are usually in pretty good shape, probably younger, most likely exercised, etc. Therefore an extra dose of Vit. C (in ascorbic acid) might work more noticeably *on their* colds and flu than many of ours. This is the thing, that doesn't mean it does *not* work or help ordinary people! It may mean the average person would likely need *more* Vit. C (if it's only in ascorbic acid it seems) and probably some other nutrients as well (as I did myself), (Vitamin C alone was not enough to subside asthma attacks altogether for myself) and organic real food and healthy habits would be great too. Well I thought, if we could figure that out and so quickly why was it not by those who conducted that trial?

Interesting isn't it. I have been dismissed so easily many times because I could not find a clinical study to show something. None that were accepted (those in conventional medicine that is) and have 'conclusive evidence' anyway. For one, I didn't just take 200 mg. Vit. C in ascorbic acid, I took 500 to 1000 at a time and more if I needed it. And for some reason, personally, I found ascorbic acid did *not* work as well as one with bioflavanoids and rosehips! I had nothing to go by at the time, but what I felt and experienced. I still wasn't into the habit of taking vitamins everyday either not seeing the importance at the time when I started, and so asthma attacks, allergies and bronchial problems would continue to return. It wasn't until I did begin taking them *regularly*, and change to a more *healthy* (non-toxic organic) diet, that asthma attacks began to rarely come along. Thus far over 4 years! (except for the 1 hour 'cold melee':) in which case just one extra C1000 (with Bioflavanoids and Rosehips:) worked great! The last time that it was pretty bad before that was during a mold condition at the end of the summer into fall here in rural Virginia then. I waited til the following year to see if it would happen again, but it didn't, nor the few following years after that and since. We're in the middle of a high allergy alert season now, and neither my son (who has had bad allergies) or myself have any problems thus far! So, my own "conclusive evidence" is it takes *regular* building up of your immune system, and *daily* vitamin taking as well. If you're still getting ill then you probably need *more* vitamins, not less, and on *a daily* basis perhaps.

So, now, which do I take being more reliable and relative? Yes, anecdotal experiences anyday! (such as those on Earthclinic.com). Some 'clinical trials' may point me in the direction but rarely will I take their "conclusive" or "inconclusive evidence" as reliable or "science" based evidence. Maybe this will give understanding of the difference between what conventional 'science based' experiments may conclude, how they're held, and how to *not* take them as the final word also! So, now I personally dismiss 'science-based' conventional clinical findings as "anecdotal"! "unscientific", unimportant and meaningless:) and nothing more!

Patti aka: rusticanecdotal:)

Kidney Stones, Olive Oil and Lemon Juice (A Non-Clinical Analysis):

Not 1, not 2, but 3 "anecdotal" testimonies for this same remedy, however it is duly noted that conventional studies say it is impossible to happen . . . hmmm

I read this first one on earthclinic.com posted it on another forum to help someone, and one responded who actually tried it and acknowledged how it worked for him also . . .

Try olive-oil and lemon juice < followed-by—> a glass of water . . .

"I have suffered intermittently from kidney stones for nearly 9 years. One was so bad I had to have surgery to remove it. Later, my grandmother was hospitalized with a kidney stone and told me about a home remedy given to her by a nurse and believe me, this really works! Mix 2 oz of olive oil and 2 oz of lemon juice, drink it straight down and follow with a large glass of water at the first sign of stone pain. The stone(s) will pass within 24 hours. I have eliminated at least 8 stones with this remedy and have not gone back to the urologist since I started taking this."

And one responded to me . . .

"I did this last month with a 7 mm stone and the <—> urologist was a little upset that it dissolved the stone. He was going to do a very expensive procedure on me that would have been both invasive and painful."

Then one other referred to it and posted it today to help someone else, having it help her son too! . . .

"I read this on here last year when my son was dealing with kidney stones and it worked. Sure can't hurt. Sorry you're going through all this, my son said it was pure hell."

My opinion is *there is* "conclusive evidence" that we're on to something here! I hope many more will be helped also with this impossible "anecdotal" remedy too. rustichealthy :)

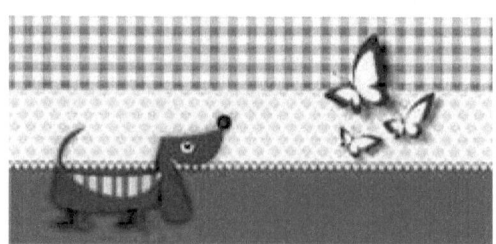

Rustic Commentary 12

Vitamins :) vs. Vaccines :/

August 2012

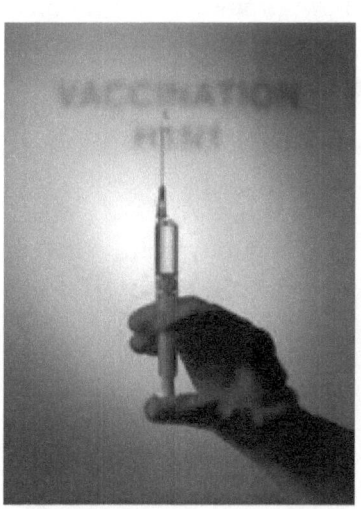

Well it's flu season again! Being on one of the conventional health and healing forums for a while, you'd think it was *always flu season*, and *always* a vaccine to be had.:/ There's always something coming around, H1N1, H1N2, H1N3 . . . pertussis/whooping cough . . . then there's swine flu, bird flu, and the latest? seal flu! I'm sure there's a "turtle flu" running around somewhere too. :) Of course it's only to coerce us to getting our vaccines. However, personally I haven't had a flu shot in years, and the last time I did have one? I had a week or so of *'flu-like' symptoms* :/ so I've opted not to get one since. Please keep in mind I have always been *very susceptible* to respiratory ailments, and if you have already read in It Takes T i m e how my first 1 hour cold/flu attack went in over 3 years:) you know already that my belief is we're all actually *vitamin deficient* (not vaccine deficient:). I did think for a while that if I went totally healthy organic, I would then no longer need vitamins, but now, (atleast from my own experience) I feel that even if I did eat total organic, as much fruits and vegetables as I can get it will not be enough for my personal conditions. Not in our changing weather (especially in cold weather for me) and availability of organic fresh healthy foods every day. For someone else it may be fine. Some have informed me that they do get perfect healthy diets (I'm assuming they have no health problems by it) and I think that's great!

Fortunately for me, we now have the technology (see, I'm not *against* 'technology', good technology that is:) to produce vitamins and nutrients available and affordable that I do need. I would look for the best quality I could find now, as close to a whole food source I could find also. For instance my Vitamin C's have bioflavanoids and wild rosehips. But now my son is telling me *organic Kamu Kamu* is the best source Vitamin C, so we're looking into that now in powder form to mix in drinks or smoothies. And, speaking of 'pandemics' such as the one in California, pertussis i.e. whooping cough, I believe is a deficiency of Vit. C (having read it's been treated with IV Vit. C successfully I then "hypothesized" it's a Vit. C deficiency) . . . perhaps in need of some other vitamins like A or omega 3's, to fight infections, as I believe they all work together more effectively too. Actually, the same for all the other flus and viruses. Instead of vaccines we may need to build up our immunity with *vitamins and nutrients* that will then *ward off* most all of these diseases. We have a *pandemic* of vitamin deficiencies! Whether you choose to get a vaccine or not I believe we may always need added nutrients, going organic as much as possible, and eliminating toxins as much as possible. This is why you won't have to be alarmed or *feel helpless* when you hear these latest threats of flu seasons and "pandemics" (a scary word in itself isn't it?). I'd always have Vitamin C's (my *stealth fav:)* around, and some of these other nutrients here that are ready willing and able for battle!:

	Apple Cider Vinegar	Ceylon Cinnamon
(a natural antibiotic)		
	Coconut Oil	Raw Honey
(great for saw throats)		
	Black Strap Molasses	Raw Bee Pollen
(a natural multi-nutrient)		
	Garlic (nature's superfood)	

Lemon Juice (alkalizes along with baking soda and apple cider vinegar), Vitamins C, D and Flax seed oil . . . And absolutely some *homemade chicken soup! (see my Rustic Healthy recipe too:)*

Before going out shopping or in public I'll usually take an extra Vitamin C and D3 also, so . . .

Get Healthy, Stay Healthy . . . Patti aka: rustichealthy :)

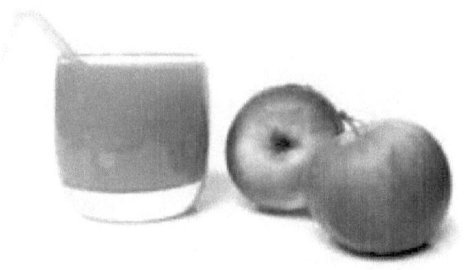

For every drug that benefits a patient, there is a natural substance that can achieve the same effect. Carl C. Pfeiffer, M.D., Ph.D.

Other Natural Antivirals?

Viruses and bacteria are the cause of many illnesses from the common cold and flu to more serious diseases such as hepatitis and meningitis, and they're everywhere and always present. While proper hygiene and sanitation are important for preventing the spread of disease many herbal remedies provide extra protection and even effective natural (less toxic) treatments . . . .

Astragalus has both antiviral and antibacterial properties. **Echinacea** is a popular herb used to prevent and treat cold and the flu. It is considered a natural antibiotic and has shown antiviral properties. **Garlic** is a powerful natural antibiotic. Its chemical component, allicin, is estimated to equal 15 standard units of penicillin! wow It is also antifungal and is used to kill parasites. **Licorice** has been shown to have anti-viral, anti-tumor and anti-inflammatory properties. **Myrrh** has been used for centuries as an antiseptic and disinfectant for wounds. Myrrh oil makes an excellent remedy for sore throats and canker sores. **Peppermint** is soothing for the stomach and neutralizes gas, but it is also an antimicrobial and antiviral.

Please remember: Vitamin supplements may have allergy affects in rare cases. Some vitamin supplements may also conflict with any medications you are taking as well. Always consult with your doctor before taking them.

===

Rustic Commentary 13

Nip it in the Bud!

September 2012

This is sort of a continuation of "Pain Management". A few days ago someone asked about natural remedy for bags under eyes. A small cosmetic issue you'd say right? I did look them up, and found a few, cucumbers, green tea bags soaked, and placed on eyes. Nice, natural, safe, even healthy! But, *this* time, I thought "Hmmm . . . I wonder if it's a 'vitamin deficiency' also?" and so typed in "vitamins for bags under eyes", and sure enough it is also a vitamin deficiency, and not just one! Vit. C, E, A, K. And so I once again got to think about my "hypothesis" that most all illnesses are a vitamin deficiency (or too many toxins). This is the importance I want to make of it. Even something as small as bags under eyes, (or a headache, heartburn as I discussed in Pain Management), or even chapped hands. Did you know chapped hands means a deficiency also? Either that *or* too many toxins again that your body is unable to process naturally and therefore deplete you of the vitamins you do get. So, lets say you have bags under your eyes? Take that as an indication that that may also mean your body is affected elsewhere that you can't see or know of, because of a lack of vitamins (or too many toxins). Or dry chapped hands? same thing. Look up natural remedies by all means! but it's not *only* bags under eyes, or only chapped hands in need of a moisturizer (or a headache or heartburn). It's a very good indication that your body is telling you something *more*. So, another part of my 'health watch' now is it is much much easier to "nip something in the bud"! A sniffle? catch it *before* it turns into a cold. That's your body saying you have something coming on that you need to be ready to tackle. Take an extra Vit. C perhaps in that case. You may hear someone say . . . "I'm fighting it" (the cold one has, or flu one is coming down with). But remember, it's not just about *your strong will* (though I am strong in the "placebo force":) and that's what conventionals allege regarding any natural whole remedy I've taken:) no, you have to give your body good effective *ammunition* to be fighting it with! i.e. vitamins and nutrients (what your body actually uses and needs to heal *itself*). Chapped hands? look up deficiency for it. Also interestingly, it's when I went organic, that I noticed my chapped hands actually stopped even in the cold blustery winter weather and have not returned as yet! I always took it as a given that I only had to find the right hand cream one day! I was taking the same nutrients as usual, however now no longer taking in *the toxins* that were in the non-organic foods. So my thinking is with that, my body is now able to *utilize* the vitamins I was taking all along in a more *effective* way now that even prevents dry skin and chapped hands, because it no longer has the toxins and "free radicals" to fight off. (And another way to save money!)

Another subject that came up recently is coffee (kind of a similar). I spoke with a friend online who would have migraines (not just a mild headache) from having just one cup of regular coffee. He had been prescribed a few supplements (magnesium being one, B12 I believe was the other). And, after a period of time he actually tried a regular cup of coffee and *did not get a migraine!*

Funny thing is my own reaction to regular coffee happens when I *stop* drinking it, I'd have a dreadful sick-day of headache and stomach upset realizing (a kind of "withdrawal" I suppose) of what I believed at the time was from the caffeine in regular coffee. So for years I've been drinking decaf, or then 'half-caf' which affected me less if I ran out so I went with it. However in my now new "organic quest", I bought organic ground coffee. Yes, caffeinated organic strong french roast coffee. I did run out of it for the second time just recently. I didn't mention it because I wanted to be sure it was true. This second time as well as the first, I actually did *not have a sick day and headache*, not even a little bit! So, now I'm wondering if it's the caffeine afterall? That it perhaps it has something more to do with the growing and process of non-organic coffee that affected me? So, when you hear of the affects of coffee consider what's being spoken of may well be non-organic coffee, (or non-organic milk, sugar . . . etc) and the growing and the process of it that may be affecting you also in a negative way.

Anyway, hope these little 'findings' help you be more aware of vitamin deficiencies for even seemingly little things, being better prepared and know the importance of perhaps fighting off things *before* they become big, and eliminating the cause or a contributing factor in the first place (toxins), by going organic also.

Patti aka: rustichealthy :)
Nipping it in the bud

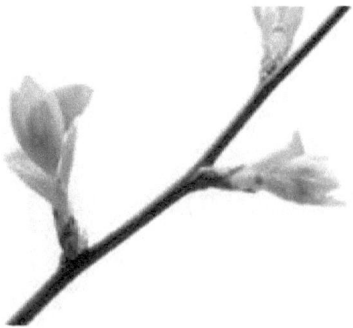

Please remember: Vitamin supplements may have allergy affects in rare cases. Some vitamin supplements may also conflict with any medications you are taking as well. Always consult with your doctor before taking them.

==

Rustic Commentary 14

Barking up the Wrong Tree (again)

October 2012

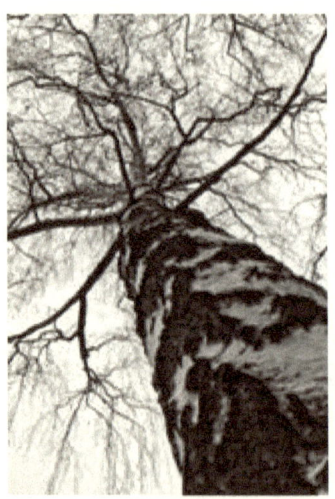

A post, on one health and healing forum stated: "FDA OKs Ultrasound System for Dense Breasts" and spoke of how amazing new technology will detect breast cancer in dense breasts, in addition to taking mammograms of course . . . . and how "37,000 women will die this year from breast cancer."

That's alarming to me, 37,000? And, the money and time put into detecting cancer, and treating it is very impressive. FDA has approved this recent technology. How well they're looking out for detection and finding treatment for breast cancer. As always "modern technology" and $ is put into more sophisticated equipment, when in my thinking the same $ could and should rather be going into more sophisticated technological ways to:

1. *Get rid of the toxins that cause the cancers* to begin with! and

2. Find other safer ways of doing things like creating safe containers, safer substances to grow food (organicly of course), safer ways to treat water, safer ways to detect and treat illness . . . including cancers.

So the post begged the question (in my mind of course), and I did ask . . .

Yet they still allow < rustichealthy > the toxins that cause it . . . why is that. (?) (and gave the link I had). And so one of my <-> trollers :) answered the following . . .

"You're either born with dense breasts <—> or you're not. Either you're big-boned or you're not. You get one parent's big nose, or you don't. Get it?"

:) to which I answered . . .

You're not born **with carcinogens . . . they < rustichealthy > come from** *Toxins* **. . . get that?** And so it went from there;)

With all the references I had given, with all the toxins mentioned, yet no care, question or concern? Why is it? How easily dismissed is it? I still do not get that. What's amazing is, the hugest deal is made of 2 or 3 dying of a virus in a remote part of the country but somehow, 37,000 people dying because of *toxins i.e. carcinogens* a year, (and many more with other types of cancers actually) is not or will not seem to be recognized as an issue! or if it is, I have not heard it ever mentioned. In the same way the media (and ny mayor) go after HFCS, once again "barking up the wrong tree!." To get to the the solution of a problem, you would have to discover what is causing it, and stop whatever it is that's contributing to it (in this case cancer and carcinogens?). Yet, to hear how easily it is dismissed by some. The *true reason* we're in such a huge health crisis in this country is because of too many dangerous carcinogenic *toxins,* actually recognized and labeled as cancer causing *carcinogens!* I don't know if I'll ever get that. We will forever be "Barking up the wrong tree" it very sadly seems to me . . . :(

Patti aka: rusticbarking :)

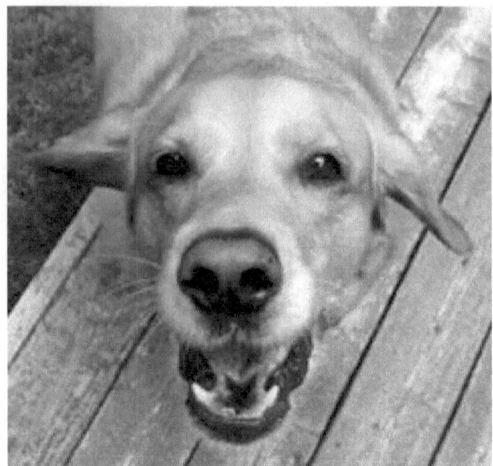

Rustic Commentary 15

Vitamin C (with Bioflavanoids & Rosehips) Still my Stealth Fav :)

November 2012

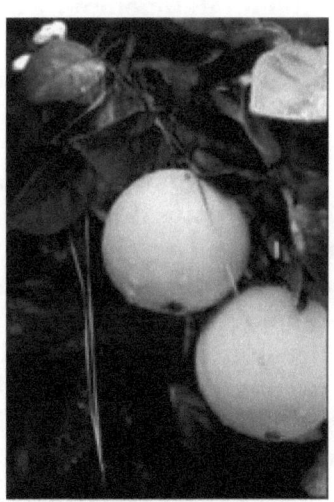

So we had another *"healthy"* debate:) today in "the Belly of the Beast:) . . . one topic on a book **"Eat to save your life", another half truth book"** . . . and the other topic **"Scare mongering to sell Water filters"** . . . though they intertwined actually. Of course vitamins came up (since I'm there:) I shared how Vitamin C with bioflavanoids and rosehips for some reason that I really didn't understand at the time when I began taking them, worked better than simple 'ascorbic acid' (the substance most clinical trials seem to use). I personally "hypothesized" that Vit C with bioflavanoids and rosehips may be closer to the original source of Vit. C than ascorbic acid and therefore more beneficial and effective. From that I was accused of being "incapable of thought and learning" and a few other things that all chimed in on, how ascorbic acid *IS* Vit. C, how I'm duped, stupid . . . etc, etc, etc. This is some of it where I began . . .

rustichealthy

I am susceptible to colds, (especially in cold weather), and, just few days ago I staved off another with an extra Vitamin C1000 (with bioflavanoids and rosehips), apple cider vinegar, honey and cinnamon . . . the 2nd time already this season. Actually this will be 4 years without a full out cold (except for one last January which lasted an hour) . . . so, I'm really not sure how 'studies' can show vitamins as ineffective "placebos" . . . but, hey, they work for me very very well! I do also take other vitamins regularly, flax seed oil, Vit. D, B Vitamins, zinc sometimes, and I try eating organic because of less pesticides, hormones, antibiotics (even courts now say should not be in them), so it seems to me the book is pretty much on the right track. It's actually my own conclusion, that most disease is a vitamin deficiency . . . sorry to disagree with the critique of the op's review of the book.

And, Dr—responded to me:

@ rustichealthy, You say you haven't had a cold in 4 years, and you attribute it to following your diet and supplement regimen. I haven't had a cold in at least 16 years, and I attribute it to NOT following your regimen, but to eating a variety of non-organic foods and avoiding supplements. I don't even take a daily multivitamin. This approach works for me! How can you possibly accuse me of being wrong? It's my own hypothesis that most diseases are not vitamin deficiencies. It would seem that my plan is 4 times as good as yours, and I have just as much evidence as you do. Are you ready to try what I recommend? Why do you think I should be ready to try what you recommend?

To which I responded:

rustichealthy: "Dr.— . . . I did try your plan, (not taking vitamins and eating non-organic:) **and I got colds 3 or 4 times a year, asthma, bronchitis, and flu. :) The difference I believe is, I am susceptible**

to them, and so I see the benefits of my plan working in that particular area. Not every one is the same . . . I understand . . . but, I was trying to give an example of vitamins working, and more specifically, not just ascorbic acid in low dose . . . that it seems the 'studies' usually go on." "I also was diagnosed with arthritis, started taking calcium supplements with magnesium and Vit. D, and no other real problems with it since . . . so, studies that say they don't work are puzzling to me."

I then tried to demonstrate how I continue to find conventional studies that are inconclusive to effects of vitamins, and yet what others actually experience when they do try vitamins . . .

rustichealthy: "Dr.— . . . ok . . . this is a study . . . that says . . . . 'At present, evidence from randomised-controlled trials is insufficient to recommend a specific role for vitamin C in the treatment of asthma. Further methodologically strong and large-scale randomised controlled trials are warranted in order to address the question of the effectiveness of vitamin C in children with asthma. And this is what one told me the other day (on another forum) . . .

and I posted what one had experienced after trying Vitamin C for herself, and how it helped her asthma also! . . .

(I continued to Dr—) **It's interesting how continually I find experiences of people (including my own) who actually try it . . . yet 'inconclusive evidence' on conventional studies.**

Then the fun begins . . . :) (*this is the Belly of the Beast remember*) and after my neglect to respond to a 'pop quiz' of a list of chemicals I was given to identify :/ since I could not label them correctly, that somehow "proves" I'm wrong about my own health experience with Vitamin C (?) . . . another poster addressed me:

****"First of all, if you are not getting your Vitamin C from ascorbic acid, I don't even know if you are getting Vitamin C at all," (?) "since ascorbic acid IS the chemical name for Vitamin C. Similarly, dihydrogen monoxide is just (pure) water, dioxygen just oxygen. DeoxyriboNucleic Acid is DNA, RiboNucleic Acid is RNA, both of which are the building blocks of all life on Earth. Good luck having a life without those. Acetylcholine is a neurotransmitter,**

responsible, among other things, for the contraction of rough red muscle cells. Without this neurotransmitter, your nervous system cannot tell a muscle to contract. Sodium Chloride is table salt. Hydrous ferric oxide is rust." (so therefore I'm wrong about vitamins and what they've done for me). Poster continued . . .

I'm not a doctor or a scientist. I have a BA in English Literature (with three hours short of a BA in Philosophy and six hours short of a Master of Fine Arts), and yet, I have managed to identify all of the chemicals listed by the participants of this thread without resorting to any online help.

You, on the other hand, have demonstrated again and again your ignorance and your basic lack of critical thinking.

:) to which I answered . . . .

********, if you ate only ascorbic acid, you'd be imbalanced adversely because it's not in it's correct natural state as it is meant to be taken along with other nutrients/fiber/juice and anything else food is comprised of . . . so therefore, taking it in a more natural surrounding would be the beneficial and preferred method imo . . . and apparently why ascorbic acid alone does *not* work or show the same benefits I've experienced, as your studies say . . . and I don't think it takes a PHD to figure that out either . . .

I was then politely asked to **"go away"** this time :) so I (tried anyway) to conclude my stay with the following . . .

My personal experience is ascorbic acid did not work as well (with my asthma attacks) as one with bioflavanoids and rosehips. That's how I concluded it may not be the best form to take and why the studies don't show it's effectiveness. It seems one needs more mgs. when it is in ascorbic acid alone in that case. That's how I know it's not as effective, and my belief that the closer to the way it's presented in nature (or replicated) the more beneficial. The only opinions the studies I've found on pubmed come to are "insufficient", or "inconclusive" evidence actually, (not conclusively saying it *Doesn't* work) which, personally, I'm glad I didn't wait another 30 or 40 years for them to perhaps come to the correct conclusion . . . finally . . . sigh . . . :) See you all another time. :)

After a few more "comments" by the others . . . Dr.—said this . . .

Dr H

To be fair, *(Thank you!:)* I think what Rustichealthy means by "ascorbic acid" is the purified ascorbic acid in a vitamin C pill as opposed to vitamin C mixed with other stuff in a "natural" source, as in rose hips. She hasn't provided any evidence that one is superior to the other, but we all generally accept the idea that it's better to get vitamins from our food rather than from a pill.

rustichealthy

"Thank you Dr. H . . . and I gave another link to back my claim that stated . . .

. . . natural vs. synthetic . . . . most sources equate vitamin C with ascorbic acid, as though they were the same thing. They're not. Ascorbic acid is an isolate, a fraction, a distillate of naturally occurring vitamin C. In addition to ascorbic acid, vitamin C must include . . . other components as shown in the figure below:

In addition, mineral co-factors must be available in proper amounts.

If any of these parts are missing, there is no vitamin C, no vitamin activity. When some of them are present, the body will draw on its own stores to make up the differences, so that the whole vitamin may be present. Only then will vitamin activity take place, provided that all other conditions and co-factors are present. Ascorbic acid is described merely as the "antioxidant wrapper" . . . . ascorbic acid protects the functional parts of the vitamin from rapid oxidation or breakdown . . .

And, what I experienced, a better result from bioflavanoids and rosehips with Vitamin C . . . . not solely ascorbic acid . . . .

. . . I won't 'trouble' you all anymore today :) have a good one . . ."

And, so, that was the end of that "episode" in the Belly of the Beast (so I thought :) . . . but, I'm happy to actually have found a link that explained and confirmed what my experience was once again. Vitamins are meant to be had in their most *natural whole food state preferably and optimally*, however, secondarily, they can be found, and had in supplement, perhaps powder form also. So, once again I stress when you look for vitamins look for as close to nature whole food source as you can for the best results. It's great when we get them in organic whole foods, however in all the varied climates and availability I do not believe this is possible on any regular basis personally.

And yes, beyond a shadow of a doubt, Vitamin C1000 *With rosehips and bioflavanoids* is *still one of* my stealth fav :)

Patti aka: rustichealthy once again another venture in . . .

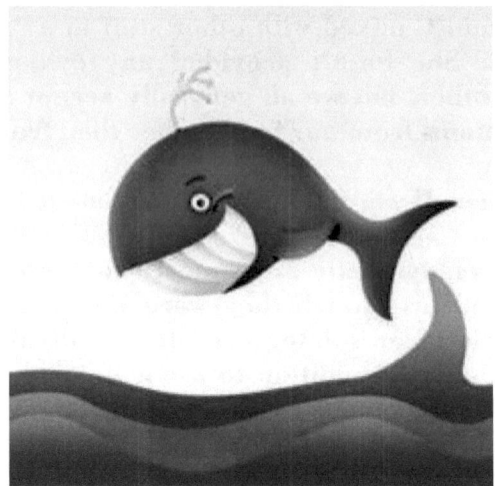

Please remember: Vitamin supplements may have allergy affects in rare cases. Some vitamin supplements may also conflict with any medications you are taking as well. Always consult with your doctor before taking them.

Rustic Commentary 16

From Fluoride to Freedom:)

November 2012

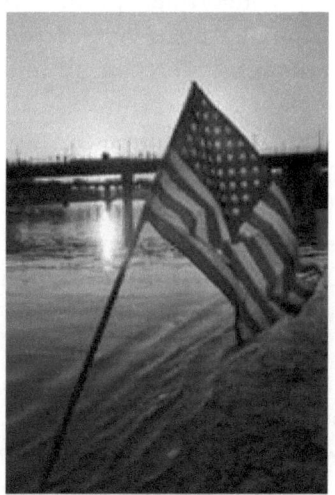

So we went from Vitamin C (with bioflavanoids and rosehips) to Fluoride to Freedom! . . . in the Belly of the Beast this week. It got to the point, after having been told what our forefathers meant (or, what they want us to believe they meant), that I figured I would post Thomas Jefferson's quotes, one who actually wrote the Declaration of Independence, and what exactly was meant by it.

Fluoride in everyone's water, and my not wanting it, meant to one that I just wanted a "customized water treatment" ummm . . . no I want *water*, not a *dental treatment* (which according to their own science means turning your teeth brown! (known as fluorosis) and that's supposed to be *harmless hmmm*) when we drink and use water. One of my arguments was, "Hey look, even if I can't provide evidence one way or the other, it's still a form of *tyranny* to force something on everyone without their personal consent". But of course in the name of "But what if one parent somewhere doesn't know how to buy toothpaste(?)" So therefore I'm being selfish and insensitive! . . . o boy . . . to which I answered . . . "What about the poor who *don't want* fluoride in their drinking water, but who *can't* afford the expensive fluoride filter?" . . . I didn't get an answer though :/

Then it went from fluoride treatment to all alternative remedies of course, and how they're all a 'scam' now and should be halted or taken control of. Meaning, vitamins, herbs, and any other 'first do no harm' remedies and people choose to invest their *own* money in for their *own* health care, according to their *own* freedom should be banned and/or taken control of by conventionals . . . For the people's own good of course! I was speechless quite a few times trying to not respond with what I felt and actually thought I was hearing. ^*((&%$##^&** :/

Seriously, it is quite disconcerting, the idea that they do believe they can actually speak for *anyone* let alone for *everyone!* I'm so happy Thomas Jefferson wrote what his thoughts were for all and any to see, to put it in correct perspective, though it seemed useless there in the Belly of the Beast. Is America, the one our forefathers fought and died for really lost now altogether? I wonder.

Here's one of my last responding comments . . .

Freedom to . . . be left alone. "Scamming" if there is scamming, is left for a Court of Law (on individual cases) . . . not by you (conventionals) . . . to determine for anyone else. That's what we have Courts for . . . .

In a country that have MILLIONS of people with differrent views and opinions of what health care is . . . the Gov should be the least to monitor what people choose to spend their own money on freely for themselves . . . the hubris of conventionals knows no bounds apparently.

It's not the same. You can choose to have whatever healthcare you want, as long as your healthcare is not infringing on my healthcare and rights . . . now you're tyrannizing my freedom, threatening to take away my free will and choice . . . or injecting toxins in my food, air and water (including fluoride) out to poison everyone actually is infringing on everyone's rights! Why you would argue for it . . . makes me wonder what it has done already . . . and,

it is no business of yours what I or anyone choose to spend their $ on!

Sorry I kind of was upset when it went to *'looking out for our pocketbooks'* . . . then a few more afterwards. One brought up the great things we got from 'big (overbearing) Gov, like Rome! . . . to which I answered . . ."slavery, gladiators and lion feeding"! . . . They kind of forgot about those 'great' feats :/

Patti aka: rustichealthy : *(from in the Belly of the Beast)* (I also question who's doing the "scaremongering"?)

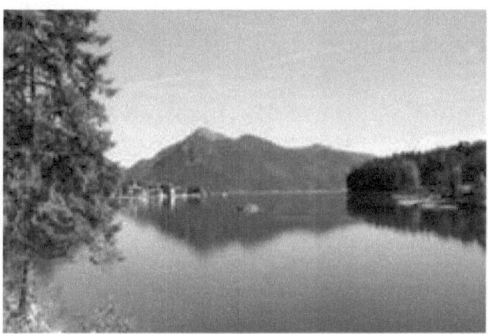

—

Here are some Jefferson quotes I posted . . . some are amazingly relative today . . .

"When the government fears the people, you have liberty. When the people fear the government you have tyranny."

Was the government to prescribe to us our medicine and diet, our bodies would be in such keeping as our souls are now. (As in 'prescribing' fluoride in all our water?).

The policy of the American government is to leave their citizens free (alone), **neither restraining nor aiding them in their pursuits.**

I think myself that we have more machinery of government than is necessary, too many parasites living on the labor of the industrious. (Back then!) That's an interesting one . . . one in the Belly of the Beast alluded to my "parasitical existence" . . . Thomas Jefferson called politicians and government officials . . . Parasites :p :) Ha!

I am not a friend to a very energetic government. It is always oppressive.

In matters of style, swim with the current; In matters of principle, stand like a rock.

The spirit of resistance to government is so valuable on certain occasions that I wish it to be always kept alive. It will often be exercised when wrong, but better so than not to be exercised at all.

The majority, oppressing an individual, is guilty of a crime, abuses its strength, and by acting on the law of the strongest breaks up the foundations of society. ("We're a Republic for as long as we can keep it" . . . the Constitution is written for the individual not the majority rule)

Were we directed from Washington when to sow and when to reap, (or what healthcare we should have?) **we should soon want bread.** (uh oh)

The price of freedom is eternal vigilance. (even in the seemingly 'small' issue like forcing fluoride in all our water)

He who knows nothing is closer to the truth than he whose mind is filled with falsehoods and errors. (Yes!)

I predict future happiness for Americans if they can prevent the government from wasting the labors of the people (spending our money) **under the pretense of taking care of them.** (!!) (Oh . . . My . . . Goodness)

I have sworn on the altar of God eternal hostility against every form of tyranny over the mind of man. (Amen)

I have never been able to conceive how any rational being could propose happiness to himself from the exercise of power over others. (me either TJ)

Most bad government has grown out of too much government.

The two enemies of the people are criminals and government, so let us tie the second down with the chains of the Constitution so the second will not become the legalized version of the first.

Sometimes it is said that man cannot be trusted with the government of himself. Can he, then, be trusted with the government of others?

A free people [claim] their rights as derived from the laws of nature, and not as the gift of their chief magistrate. (i.e. government officials and politicians i.e. "Parasites" :p :)

The right of self-government does not comprehend the government of others.

An elective despotism was not the government we fought for. (tell it TJ!)

It is better to tolerate that rare instance of a parent's refusing to let his child be educated, than to shock the common feelings by a forcible transportation and education of the infant against the will of his father. (i.e. public education i.e. indoctrination)

The natural progress of things is for liberty to yield and government to gain ground. (. . . and where are we at now in this great America that our forefathers and children paid in blood for?) :(
Thomas Jefferson Famous Quotes

~~~~~~

How *"healthy"* is fluoride? . . .

The chemicals used for fluoridation are *not high purity, pharmaceutical quality products*. Rather they are byproducts of aluminum and fertilizer manufacturing and contain a high concentration of toxins and heavy metals such as arsenic, lead and chromium. All proven to be carcinogens.

One of my last posts was:

"Freedom of Speech *is dangerous* only to those who wish to silence it." :) Did someone say that already? if not . . . you can put that down as one of mine :) rustichealthy . . . on my last "excursion" inside "the Belly of the Beast"

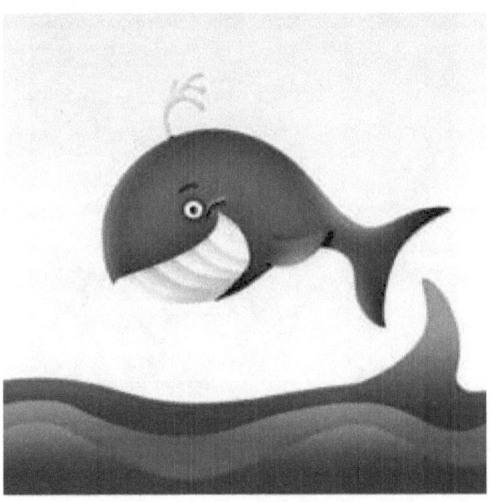

"Government does not solve problems, it subsidizes them. A government bureau is the nearest thing to eternal life we'll ever see on this earth." President Ronald Reagan

===

Rustic Commentary 17

On the Cold War Front

January 2013

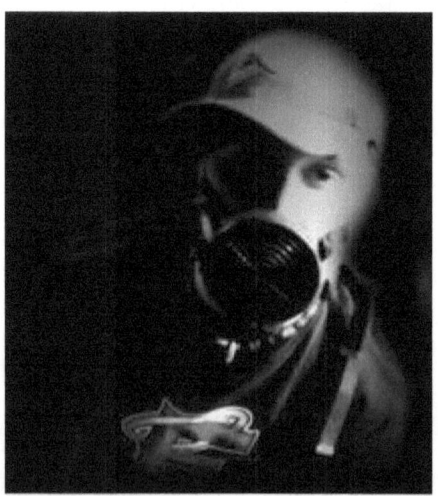

Well, we've been in discussion on this recently . . .

I always believed it was simply accepted that when it's cold weather, your immune system is brought down, having to deal with the cold as well as everything else. I know that's what I've experienced personally for many years, and I still am susceptible in the cold. I didn't know the details or studies of it however, nor did I realize it was disputed. Naturally our bodies were not meant for 'cold' weather. How do I *know* that? Because, we need to wear extra warm apparel in the cold weather! We (or some anyway) may be able to adapt a little better of course, and may have stronger "immune systems" as well . . . probably younger people, or more in shape and active people (as in the military or an athlete). But, nevertheless cold weather does bring down immune systems in most everyone sooner or later anyway. No one can stay out in the cold improperly dressed for hours and hours without being affected by it in some way. I believe cold and flu viruses are contracted more so in the winter and cold weather months because people's immune systems are down having to also fight off the cold temperatures to the body (that we're not meant for). So you may ask, "But Rustic, what about summer colds"? I thought of that too and, what I observed carefully is, it's usually when I am in a cold air-conditioned store, near a cold air conditioner, or in and out of cold water that's when my immune system comes down, and I end up either (in the past) with a bad summer cold, or now having to take extra vitamins so the cold does not develop (as my "Nip it in the Bud" or "Vitamins vs Vaccines" commentaries explain) and as I've covered in my last cold experience. What we need are *nutrients* to build our immunity to them, both colds and flus (in particular in cold weather). Cold and flu viruses are everywhere, and that is the one and only sure thing to fight them off. Vaccines even they say are only 63% sure (this year it was said less than that actually) and then perhaps only of a few certain flu viruses or what is designated as 'dangerous' for that year. I say, "Yep . . . they're barking up the wrong tree again!" It's vitamins, nutrients and healthy (organic) whole food, and *yes keeping warm*, dry and protected (as most all moms knew) as much as possible that will prevent many a cold or flu.

A study in Wales proved **"drops in temperature to the body can cause a cold to develop. Out of 180 vollunteers half had their feet immersed in ice cold water for 20 minutes."** (It would only take one minute for it to affect me actually). **"The other 90 in tests during the common cold "season" sat with their feet in an empty bowl. During the next four or five days, almost a third of the chilled volunteers developed cold symptoms—compared to just 9 percent in the control group, the scientists said."**

The researchers said that common colds were more prevalent in the winter than the summer, and this could be related to an increased incidence of chilling causing more clinical colds. But they also suggested that another explanation could be that our noses are colder in the winter.

My continued "advice" is, keep dry and warm, *and* don't forget to take extra vitamins too during "cold and flu season". :)

This is now my personal go-to protocol at the very first sniffle or sign of a cold/flu:

Apple cider vinegar (antiseptic, alkalizes) followed by or mixed in water

Honey (antibacterial healing properties)

Ceylon cinnamon (sprinkled on top of the honey) a powerful natural antibiotic and an extra Vitamin C 1000 (with bioflavanoids and rosehips my stealth fav) a natural antihistamine and immunity builder. and, a hot cup of organic black tea, or nice homemade chicken soup! (with healthy organic vegetables of course) for added nutrients and help.

Three vitamin/nutrients to have for the ready:)

Vitamin C . . . . has been demonstrated to have a strong anti-viral effect. In high doses, vitamin C neutralizes free radicals, helps kill viruses, and strengthens the body's immune system.

Vitamin D . . . . The best source of vitamin D is sun exposure. In lieu of sunlight, food and supplements are your next best option. D3 is the natural source. (D2 is synthetic) **and Zinc . . . It has been shown that zinc lozenges or syrup taken early in the course of a cold can shorten its duration and severity.**

And to be "fair and balanced", here is part of what was given to counter my own thinking

"On the contrary, cold weather appears to stimulate the immune system . . ." Researchers examined the immunological responses to cold exposure and found that acute cold exposure, such as going outside without a jacket, actually appears to activate the immune system." This occurs in part by increasing the levels of circulating norepinephrine, one of the body's hormones, which works as a natural decongestant."

My personal consideration to that is, your body may indeed have limited natural defense, and perhaps in those who already have a healthy strong immune system. However, if you're getting colds in cold weather then your immunity is not strengthened afterall. You need to stay warm, (and add extra nutrients to build your immunity still). However, it is up to you to consider how to deal with your own colds and flu of course :)

"I report, you decide" :) . . . reporting from the Cold War Front Lines
Patti: aka rustichealthy

Flu Vaccine Effectiveness Update

A little update on this years 'effectiveness' of the flu vaccine . . .

A U.S. government analysis of this season's flu vaccine suggests it was effective in only 56 percent of people who got the shot, and it largely failed to protect the elderly against an especially deadly strain circulating during flu season.

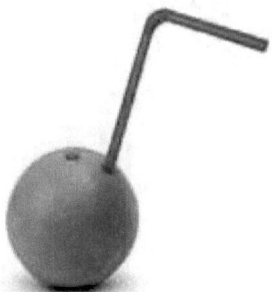

Rustic Commentary 18

Dealing with "death trolls"

February 2013

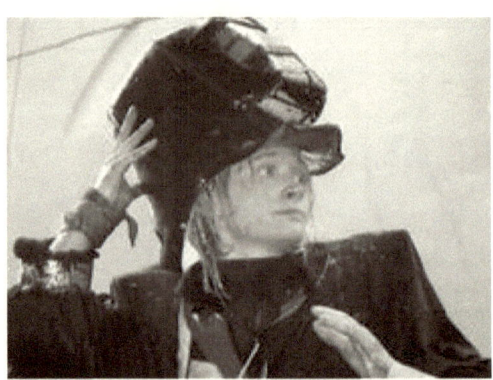

It has been dark days on the health and healing alternatives forum. Con(ventional) trolls seem to have made it their home now :/ So, it's been reminiscent of the days of old (last year) in the conventional health forum, where I was "attacked" relentlessly (as crystbear). This was a difficult, actually unexpected long "battle" recently in the alternative forum, when one came in looking for alternative help for pain. A 42 year old who had an advanced case of cancer, myself admittedly not knowledgeable of it all of course, but it had to do with his kidneys and bladder and was now spreading. At first in thinking of how to help him naturally with pain I suggested some natural pain relief with cinnamon (knowing someone was helped with it and his fibromyalgia and bad arthritis see Testimonials) but I then asked did he want some other alternatives with his conditions, but he was talking to another. Then, a few began to speak of and administer "palliative" care and how a hospice could help him with his 'end of life' situation, and just reading them actually made me sicker by the minute. Literally sick to my stomach (if I remember how one feels that sick since I haven't for a long while:) That's when I decided to atleast reach out again. This is where I entered:

********. . . you sound young . . . you have plenty < rustichealthy > of life ahead! There are things that can help. How do you know alternatives won't work until you try? . . . Try baking soda? flax oil? vitamins? there's so many things, even for your condition that conventional medicine says won't work, but they do for others. I hope you consider it :)

I asked him how old he was, (he sounded young to me) and yes, he is just 42! I said that's young! and he said yes "Way young"! so I began telling him about some others, as the 79 year old in 3rd stage lung cancer helped with flax seed oil and cottage cheese, (on Testimonials also), and about another and his help with 4th Stage prostate cancer and was sent home to die, yet turned around with something as simple as baking soda and molasses. He said along the way (in between all the interference and "attacks" by the "death trolls" (so I ended up labeling them), acting as if *my* attempting to give *some hope was "evil"*, but that he was open to different things now and going out with his 'boots on'!, and I said, "well, this is the way!".

In this "altercation", there were 'complimentary' alternatives administering 'end-of-life' comfort, and actually a few other conventionals who had advanced cancer calling me a 'dolt', cruel, clueless for giving *false hope'*, and more. It was rather surreal to say the least. You would think, (in a normal audience that is), people would say, well, it doesn't sound harmful! baking soda, molasses, flax oil, apple cider vinegar! if it helps a little, wouldn't it 'be nice' to give it a try? No! I had these Con(ventional) Trolls literally screaming, insulting, (one wanted to reach into his/her computer and smack me! if they could!). I know, you had to be there. It was amazingly like an alternate universe. Here's just some of the comments, the first few were mine:

This is just one that wrote to my son . . . < rustichealthy > (I gave the incident of the 79 year old and stage 3 lung cancer, and how cottage cheese and flax seed oil was helping him) . . .

This is the flax oil treatment. (link) **It's important to try detoxing . . . what I mean is, eating organic grown fruits/ vegetables . . . and taking nutrients like spirulina and chlorella.**

And, just fyi . . . try washing with < rustichealthy > baking soda and water any rashes, lesions that are on your skin. Apply apple

cider vinegar and water (if it doesn't burn too bad) . . . or you can simply apply Coconut Oil . . . it's amazing stuff . . . all three of those things are. Buy Organic ACV and coconut oil . . . with less toxins.

And, just as a basic . . . < rustichealthy > I hope you read this and the other info . . . start taking a few basic supplements . . . B Complex, C1000 and D3 . . . I'd say atleast 5000 . . . I'd say more, maybe others know and can help with that. I am praying and hoping for you hon. rustichealthy

(This is to someone who had no other advice other than pain remedies and about some "hospices" until the end.)

This is where the "trolls" entered and "battle" began . . . (I knew I was asking for it btw) the typical responses I've gotten on any natural home remedy or nutrients I've given have been trashed, dashed or mocked, but this was in particular strong . . .

Find your off button. § <—>

You are a dolt. A terminally ill person does <—> not have plenty of life ahead as you say. I would reach through my computer and smack you if I could. Your ramblings are one thing but you are downright insensitive and moronic. (o boy)

The feeling is mutual actually :) < rustichealthy > You really have no clue what is possible, and you're a typical 'death panel' conventional.

I am a terminally ill person you a*******. <—>(no way to know this) There I called you another name, and you deserve it. I'm not a '"death panel"' conventional, I'm a dying person. That is something you have no personal experience at being so just stfu.

(That kind of took me back).

Then I'm sorry . . . I had no idea . . . < rustichealthy > how could I? If you possibly could . . . read what I'm telling **********, and hope you try it. Peace.

I told you I DONT WANT TO HEAR IT STFU § < YOU-READ-IT > All cancer is not curable. It sounds <—> like this poster is seeking palliative care.

Well . . . that's what conventionals say. < rustichealthy > We want to see vinyltap out of pain And healed . . . even of this cancer.

We'd like to see that, too. <—> But baking soda and charcoal aren't going to help him.

Well I don't think you know that. § < rustichealthy >

NEITHER DO YOU, SHUT IT <—> When you get cancer, please return here and tell us all about how you are curing yourself. Until then shut up about it. I am not referring to Basal Cell Skin Cancer, I'm talking about Stage 4 cancer. And if you dare to tell me you'll never get cancer because of your vit. c and organics I am going to personally write to Craig and have him take you down.

Maybe this isn't a good place for you < rustichealthy > if it upsets you this much . . . sorry . . . but I hope you try some of the things I'm telling ****** anyway. Peace again.**

You are being cruel beyond belief, stop it now. § <->

—

Wow, so, I'm trying to help this young man and I'm called "cruel beyond belief" . . . keep in mind this is an alternative forum. And these are remedies tried and succeeded on others with advanced cancer! If hearing about "alternatives" is so upsetting to some of these posters, why do they come there . . . not sure I'll understand that.

This was the young man's last post to me on this thread, *and thankfully* he got it . . .

Much Thanks. <********> I do appreciate all input. I'm not above researching new avenues. You've brought up couple treatments I've read up on already, and a few new ones. That's the whole point, getting more info. I've aleady found that what works for others, hasn't for me. So I believe the opposite must also be investigated(ie. what doesn't seem to work on others, may work for me). I have nothing to lose.

Absolutely they will help . . . < rustichealthy > just try those three topical applications alone . . . baking soda/applecider vinegar and coconut oil for your rashes etc. every day . . . and take them . . . internally . . . everyday . . . vitamins too. This is Vern's video . . . if you haven't seen it . . . (link)

This is for kidney stones . . . it may have a good general effect on your kidney and bladder too . . . (link)

This is the cottage cheese and flax seed oil diet: (link)

**********. . . you said you want to go out < rustichealthy > with your boots on! well . . . this is the way! You won't be drugged, you'll be Helped, I believe Healed., but, definitely you can go out with your boots on! I love to hear that! God bless hon.**

Well, the trolls that continued their attack and mocking, I ended up designating each one a "Death Troll" . . . one a Stupid "Death Troll" :) . . . the one who actually called flax seed oil, baking soda and apple cider vinegar DANGEROUS Misinformation! . . . ?? to one who was dying and had *no other hope otherwise?* . . . Dangerous Misinformation? . . . really? . . . sad and amazing! What kind of mind says a thing like that? I didn't know what else to say to that and ended from there.

Of course I couldn't *guarantee* anything and the young man knew and understood that! But at least he has a chance and some hope now! And will actually look up the things I mentioned for himself. The one thing, well a few things I am happy about in this is that I happened to be there for him and that he responded, was listening and will try! (Rendering the "death trolls" in this 'attack' powerless) and that there are others reading in forum, and perhaps are getting help also. I ask that you all keep this young man in prayer also.

I was totally drained from this . . . and then in another post the next day one conveyed this to me:

Go Rustic!!!!!! <—>

Rustic thanx for all your support to all those who are very grateful you're here, and sincerely and serenely interested in real help!

THX for sticking-up and trying to keep this form healthy!

THX for bringing attention to all the conTROLLS, and all your effort to get *** ***** to put all the drug pushing disrupts in their place!**

One more thing . . . I, and a few others, over the yrs have learned to use our handles sparingly in order not to feed the conTROLLers, and be the most benefit to the ppl coming to the forums for real help.

There are a few of us watching you (on your side), I share e-mails from (************) and (*************), they have been around for yrs, never use their handles anymore, and don't hang out in the forums much anymore but when we are here, we support you!Rustic thanx for all your support to all those who are very grateful you're here, and sincerely and serenely interested in real help!

Thank you ********** :) < rustichealthy > I am so happy to hear there are more 'out there', I did notice a few <->'s giving such great intelligent advice and help, and I wondered who they were!! Nooow I know!! :) . . . I understand now what you mean by using my nic sparingly in order to help . . . I've just begun to do that too . . . (not this time unfortunately)! . . . but, I am so glad to get things out here for others to be helped . . . . Thank you so much for telling me you're here, and the others . . . it really means more than you know . . .

I hope all and any one of you will look up also some of the things I've mentioned here. At whatever stage you are at and all seems to be hopeless too.

Patti aka: rusticdealing with the "death trolls"

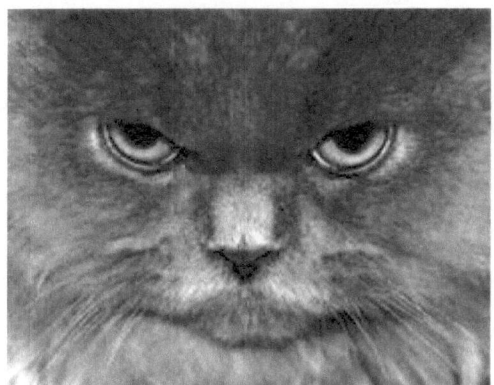

Rustic Commentary 19

A few Thank you's very much Appreciated

February 2013

After a few *more* difficult days on an alternative health forum, having to deal with quite a few 'greys', known as "trolls", who are constantly after me for everything I do and say. I happened to talk with my son about it, and said "I do hope there are others perhaps reading, and maybe some are getting help out of this" . . . and then, a very nice poster said following along with a musical note and a big THANK YOU . . .

"rustichealthy—thank you for your <***************> wonderful contribution to this and the other H&H forum!!!!
You help so many ppl and are sincere from your heart about caring about ppl and giving real help to all.
I'm glad the allopathic medicine trolls haven't run you out of this, these forums!! I saw yesterday, where last handle said s/he will give you all his/her plus points, I also will support you and give you many plus points for all your best post and whatever I have left before I log out!!"

"Wow . . . Thank you so much :) < rustichealthy > (this actually brought me to tears! :*) I don't know what to say! (a little unusual for me!) ;) I hoped others were being helped, but, honestly, I really didn't know . . . I am so so surprised! for you to do this! I am more than happy to be here . . . so glad you appreciate my contribution :)) . . . It is overwhelming sometimes, so I appreciate Every Green Point You Give!! :)) You're such a dear to post this, and I will save it and keep it forever in my heart!! :) God Bless . . . Thank You so much for being there! and doing this again . . . rustichealthy :)"

and then one other . . .

"Looking over your history rustichealthy <—> I also must say you do a very fine job taking care of your health & being healthy and responsible for your health, and you clearly care about ppl & helping ppl !!
I support you 100%!
I'm on your side!!!!!!!
I've used up all my points today, but in the future I will shower you with many plus points!
The world needs more ppl like you!!!! Thank You!!!!!!!!!"

:) That is all I wish and hope out of all of this. That others are helped too, as I have been with healthy organic food and natural helps and remedies! This was very touching to me. Even my son was so surprised also that someone actually took the time to respond with the above! (the posts included large THANK YOUs and pictures) May many more be helped and have hope too. Hey, it's Valentine's Day soon . . . and these are my first Valentines :)

Patti aka: rusticthankyou :*)

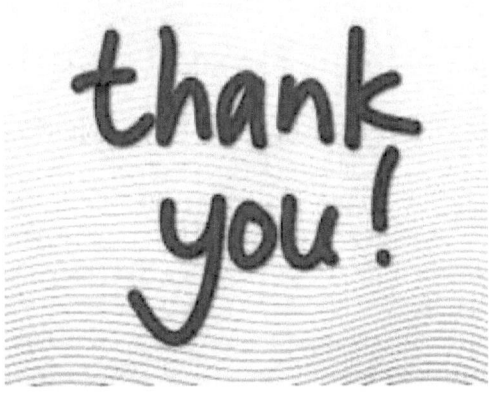

Rustic Healthy 20

On Defending Omnivores (taking on the Vegans :)

March 2013

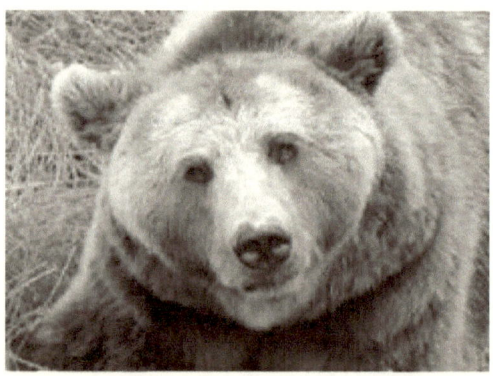

Well, I happened to take a trip over to "Veganville" (a forum for vegans) this time a week or so back back to originally garner support against CAFO's, and thought I'd recount my experience here, and some interesting things I found out about some vegans, at least in Veganville anyway :) My first response was to one who top posted this "Food for Thought" . . .

Food for Thought

I just found out something fascinating Scientists have discovered from fossil evidence that the first Dinosaurs were vegans, vegetarians:

In fact the the only dinosaur that survived the great mass extinction 250 million years ago which killed 95% of all Life on Earth was Lystrosaurus: a little puppy of a dinosaur who was a vegetarian. In fact Lystrosaurus is the ancestor of all mammals . . . So we humans originally came from a VEGETARIAN DINOSAUR. All the meat eating dinosaurs went extinct. This means that all meat eaters will also go extinct while we vegetarians will be doing just fine."

. . . and so my first response in "Veganville" was . . .

"Does that mean . . . fox and chicken too? . . . hmmmm . . . <rustichealthy > they're meat-eaters too! . . .

While living at a ranch several years ago, I was awoken at around 2 a.m. The terrorized wild screeching of one of the free range roosters, who used to walk freely among the grass with his friends, picking up bugs and worms swallowing them whole. Living and working in NYC, we were used to the screeching of sirens and trains, but not this. It was a happy life (pity the bugs and worms who had a life of their own albeit). He usually flew up in the trees at night like his friends as well, but, didn't do so for some reason on this awful, awful night of terror in the country, no one knows why. A fox now had him in his jaws, carrying him around and around around the house, screeching and fluttering, over and over and over until the poor rooster gave in and finally died, in the jaws of the fox, ending up being a tasty meal for the fox though. It was a terrifying incident, but, everything ecologically, is for a reason and necessity, and everything unfortunately dies at some point in time, whether it end up on a dinner plate, or in the jaws of a predator. No, it is not always "humane", no it is not always without suffering and loss, but it is the means of sustenance and survival. It is . . . the *"Circle of Life."* I would choose to have humane treatment of all animals, ending quick and painless as possible, having them lived a happy and decent free life as much as possible too. A free range organic happy life. I believe we can all agree on that. :)"

Well . . . I suppose that wasn't the best recount to straight out put in a Vegan forum :) another vegan spoke:

"you're asking vegans to approve of your meat? really??? pov test—how do you think a vegan would respond to this?"

"I'm asking the op if meat eaters all die out . . . < rustichealthy > and since fox and chickens are meat eaters too (chickens eat bugs and worms) . . . then that would mean they would die out too . . . according to his 'wish' . . . just wondering if he thought of that? Why?"

"your words: *   *   * "It is . . . the "circle of life." I would choose to have humane treatment of all animals, ending quick and painless as possible, having them lived a happy and decent free life as much as possible too. A free range organic happy life. I believe we can all agree on that. :)" and you post this on a VEGAN forum?"

"yes . . . and? < rustichealthy > we can all agree on humane treatment I think :)"

"why do you think people become vegan?" §<**>**

"Not sure, other than you were taught to feel < rustichealthy > guilt, one way or another, over killing even for sustenance. even to kill a fly, mosquito? Not too many thrive on killing on purpose . . . I don't know too many people, I don't know Anyone actually, who like killing for no reason. Will you defend yourself if an animal . . . dog, wolf, bear . . . comes after you? Or do you also believe you should simply be their meal for the day? I guess I would like to know some things about being vegan. yes"

"try harder"§ <**>**

:) The point I was trying to make was almost all of nature is not 'humane', and if he (the Top Poster) was thinking all carnivorous/omnivorous people and animals would die off it would also mean the fox and the chicken too! along with lions, tigers, bears, alligators . . . etc. etc. etc. etc. etc.! then ***** entered again . . . :

"You're talking about the circle of DEATH not LIFE—The point to being a vegetarian is simple:
In every mass extinction: all the top predators go extinct while the ones down the LOWEST on the food chain have a very good chance of survival. In any mass extinction: humans who eat meat will go EXTINCT: end of story. The human species is at the TOP OF THE FOOD CHAIN: thus it will be wiped out without question.
But . . . BUT! . . . the humans who do NOT eat meat are NOT at the top of the food chain: they share the vegetation around

them with other vegetarian animals and thus have a much better chance for survival.

The only mass extinction which could kill off a VEGETARIAN or VEGAN human is if every blade of grass and every tree and plant went extinct also and that has never happened so far. Chickens are NOT vegetarians or vegans. Nor are foxes. IN a mass extinction both of them will automatically go extinct . . . .

The point is:: it pays not to be at the top of anything because then you are a target to be toppled off your pedestal, and the chances are you will not last long. If you are down at the BOTTOM of the cycle of LIFE: then you will have the BEST chance of survival.

In other words: the entire concept of civilized winning is a fallacy. All the biggest mass murderers will go extinct

JUST LIKE THE DINOSAURS
While vegans will be doing just fine thank you very much to which I responded :)

The chickens have to eat bugs and worms to < rustichealth > Live, the fox have to kill chickens to Live . . . it's both, but, it is to Live ultimately. And, most humans kill or eat meat to Live . . . not because they Like killing, or the dastard inhumane treatment on CAFOs. In any case, I am hoping we can at least agree on that. But, it seems vegans have gone venomous now . . . it's showing. You have a huge imagination though . . . very impressive and vulnerable it seems to any and all made up tales it seems. to which **** responded:

You keep on using emotional words like 'venomous' You have a lot of anger issues. (I didn't think I had 'anger' issues? ok sometimes dealing with trolls:) **Killing you is not a matter of emotion. 8) I would kill you like a chicken kills a bug: without any hate or venom.** (this I would consider an 'anger' issue:/ **You do understand this don't you? that's what you do also. No hard feelings.** (yes I understand,::gulp::, no "hard feelings":) to which I responded touching something of mental problems . . . to which ******* responded . . .

I have no mental problems whatsoever you're a bug that needs to be killedYou're in favor of this detached attitude towards killing you have the detached attitude of killing animals as if they are bugs I am just returning the favor

Ok, I hadn't realized how far some were going with vegan belief! I spoke on my commentary Vegan/Vegetarian or Organic Omnivore how I completely respect one's own belief, and how they lived it out, such as in veganism, if that is how they view things, that is how they choose to live, then I respect that! I was hoping it was mutual, not so sure now :) In any case, one other vegan intervened and shared how yes, there were some 'extreme' thought vegans, however, his own belief is from his teaching, to respect all life, and simply lived it out for himself. As mine is, to "live and let live", vegan, vegetarian or omnivorous. on another thread I said:

Earth will probably be overrun with < rustichealthy > bugs and worms then! hmmmm

Be carefull what you wish for :) § < rustichealthy >

IF . . . If man did not tamper with domestic creatures, the wild ones would balance out just fine. Why mutilate, torture, and murder other creatures, since there is no noble purpose to it? What is a natural remedy for pin worms? How about tape worm? Some of the disturbed trolls around here appear to have advanced cases of those, so much so it has affected their minds. One, I believe may be suffering from advanced degenerative syphlis, that he contracted from a snakebite. What is the home remedy for that? We'd like to get them patched up and on their merry way."

and I said:

"Exactly! . . . I agree . . . didn't I agree with . . . < rustichealthy >

"Why mutilate, torture, and murder other creatures, since there is no noble purpose to it? " . . . sustenance and survival are different . . . maybe you didn't read my story there? :)"

"what's your definition of ANIMAL RIGHTS?" § <**>**

"They should be treated as humanely as possible < rustichealthy > why? I don't believe it's inhumane to kill for sustenance and survival."

"you don't need to kill animals to survive" § <**>**

"That's your belief, not mine. < rustichealthy > You choose to be a vegan, I respect that. Just as long as you don't force it on everyone else . . . that's where problems come in I think :)"

"you're forcing your carni beliefs on vegans" § <**>**

"Not at all . . . I do believe quite the opposite < rustichealthy > though :)"

"you're in our house. show some respect" § <**>**

"your nic is not sounding appropriate < rustichealth > little by little to me. Perhaps veganevil . . . or veganforce . . . or veganfascist . . . Just an observation now . . . don't take it ballistically please :)"

"y r u in a vegan forum?" <****>

"To show not all are for inhumane treatment < rustichealthy > of animals, (I believe in free range humane living and quick humane killing). And, to raise awareness of organic food also, whether one is vegan/vegetarian or omnivore. :)"

"IN that case we <******> have the right to kill you as quickly and humanely as possible: Slicing your throat while you are hanging upside down by one foot in a hook should do it"**

::::Gulp::::

It's a good thing this is the internet! There are some things to consider. Humans need omega 3s, and B12, which are readily found in fish and beef and eggs as I understand. And, not too many in history of civilization were vegetarian, not sure if any were actually 'vegan'. Vegans take a processed 'nutritional yeast' for one of their sources today, however, I don't see how it could have been plentiful before this, so, I would question if man were meant for and made originally to be 'vegan' as they were trying to allege. That's still not satisfactorily answered. I do believe man was made to be omnivorous from almost the very beginning anyway, right after "the fall" perhaps, when Abel had a herd of sheep! Why would one have a herd of sheep in a warm climate if not for meat as well? That would be my question and line of thinking anyway. In any case, it was an interesting few visits. I had other questions, like "What would "Veganville" look like? Bears, wolves, fox, chickens all running free?" "Were there limits set?" "How would they set those limits?" "What did they do about ants and roaches in the house?" Things like that. It was fun too. The Sheriff and another ******** came over to visit Alternatives as well (the Sheriff was originally informed he was "out of his 'jurisdiction'", however it was allowed as he was "conducting an investigation" (on me :) after that . . . and I was even invited back to Veganville! albeit so I could be 'shredded' . . . but, well, I took it as well-meaning anyway :)
Patti aka: "rusticomnivorous organicus" :)

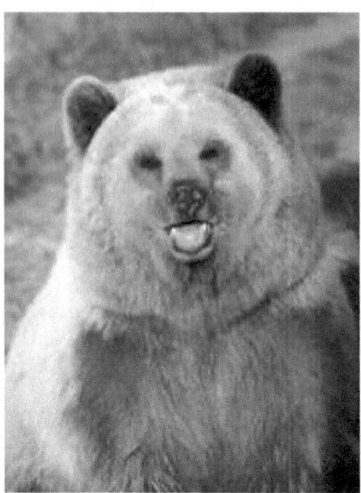

"Bears are *omnivores* too ya know!":)

Rustic Commentary 21

The New Snake Oil

March 2013

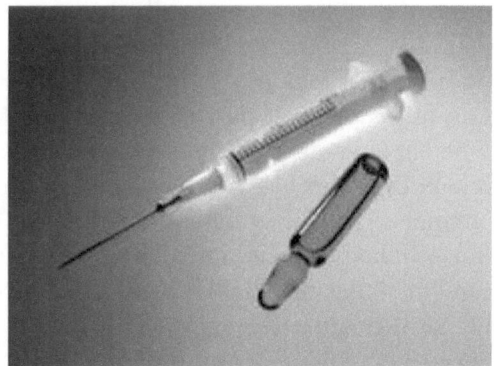

Bad "Science" and the New Snake Oil i.e. Quackery :/

Unfortunately, what may have started out with great intentions is now (in my opinion anyway) part of the seriously great problems we have today in *healthcare* and running the cost up for everyone too. Things that do not belong in the human body, introduced, that may be helping one thing, but harming in other ways. Then of course, the same who created the first 'remedy' now create another remedy (to remedy the first remedy's side effects which are sometimes worse then the original problem and so on). As I've described earlier in another chapter, a 'vicious cycle'. I still believe most in the medical profession believe they are administering 'health' the best they know how, at least I believe the majority are, but

I'm hoping some will start to see what is happening and think again what they are prescribing and ascribing to. Many of these substances, actually *known carcinogens, labeled as 'carcinogens', causing cancer themselves,* yet somehow overlooked.

We knew and heard how bad antibiotics were for many years (I remember over 30 years at least) yet they've only been increased in usage and dosage not only in medicine, but in the foods we eat every day. (remember "What Do We Get?") Steroids, something I had to use for my asthma, was very carefully prescribed and administered, only in extreme circumstances, yet today it seems they are readily used for other things that I am stunned about! I had this part on the home page, but it's grown so much I decided to make it's own page too, and this last commentary. Not only that, but it's such a downer I didn't like it there either. (Don't worry! there's still good news and good medicine!). These are things I've only come across in this last year. Once again, no I am not a doctor or health professional, but my common sense and experience says artificial synthetic substances have very little use in place of healing, at least not on an *everyday basis*, not since natural body friendly nutrients and vitamins have been discovered, that I know personally have very great results as do so many others! It also depends on the source and looking for the most whole food source is best. Just look at the Testimonials for just a few! I love giving help and hope to people, but part of it is to stop taking in the 'bad medicine' that may be causing much of the problems and ailments we have, and to stop the 'vicious cycle' at least for yourself and perhaps your loved ones. Many are convinced, and have convinced others, that nutrients and vitamins (things that our body needs and thrives on actually) are "snake oil", "quackery" and/or "placebos"!. That is what I've usually heard. Unfortunately, I believe it is quite the contrary! Vaccines now being forced on nurses or they lose their jobs?! When did this become such an issue? The vaccines themselves *actually bring down the immune system* to fight off disease itself, yet people are now compelled to take them (one nurse ending up in emergency after one), and amazingly, the cold and flu situation only seems to get worse and worse each year :/

There is Still Happy News and Good Medicine!

To sum up, and to put it simply, my whole "healthy strategy" . . . is to get as few toxins in and around us, be it through a good water filter, (fluoride filter if you have it added in your water) using natural non-toxic even healthy things like baking soda for cleaning aids and eating less chemical filled foods, by *going organic!* I try for mostly *organically grown* food as possible, and we look for non-toxic "do no harm" remedies as much as possible. I take vitamins and nutrients everyday now (as I find I do need them) and I take more if I need them also. Before going out in public, in cold weather, I'll take an *extra Vit. C.* (remember "Nip it in the Bud" and "Vitamins vs. Vaccines" :) and some other wholesome home remedies. There is really no "one size fits all" of course and your body is different than anyone's, as is your environment and diet, so those are just some basics that I've used. You may not need any! You're getting all the nutrients you may need in a healthy organic diet (7-9 servings of healthy whole foods) and that's super! For me (thus far) they're working great. We have some simple home remedies in the house and are amazed at their benefits (for just about anything it seems) the following five: (Organic) Applecider Vinegar, Blackstrap Molasses, Coconut Oil, Baking Soda, and Cinnamon!

Remember it really matters very little what stage or age you're at! There is a *lot* of help and hope! Once again see **Testimonials** and how a 79 year old is getting help for his 3rd stage lung cancer! (just for one). Anyway, I only wanted to end up with something hopeful here too.

Wishing you and your families a very Healthy, Happy 2013 the rest of!
Patti aka: RusticHealthy!! :)
"An apple a day . . ."

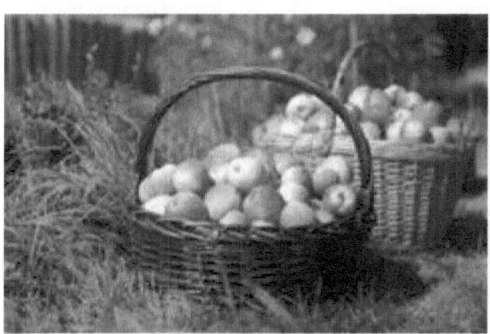

Please remember: Vitamin supplements may have allergy affects in rare cases. Some vitamin supplements may also conflict with any medications you are taking as well. Always consult with your doctor before taking them.

Rustic Healthy "Anecdotal" Testimonials

"Let Food be thy Medicine . . ."

~~~~~~~~~~~~~~~~~~~~~~~~~~~~

I've shared how I find "anecdotal" experience much more relevant and reliable then most any other clinical studies personally! These are only a few of what I felt were interesting testimonials I found and/or were given to or brought to my attention in this last year so I thought I would share them here. To me they're compelling and uplifting to see the possibilities and helps when there were none otherwise! All of them are anonymous as I have no way of contacting them personally. Just remember everyone is unique, and they may or may not work for you . . . but! there's always something else natural and healthy to look up and find for yourself too!

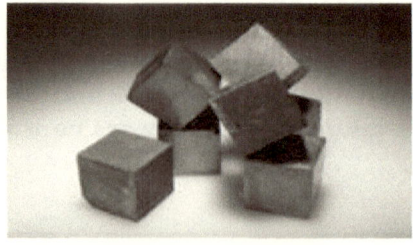

Iron Deficiency and Restless Leg Syndrome

Iron "cured" mine

I've had this for perhaps 10 years. I got so bad that I had many sleepless nights but also had leg cramps (calves) all day as well. I started researching vitamins and realized that I'd been a vegetarian for years previous. One summer day when I could hardly feel my lower legs I took 17 mg of iron at about 1 PM. Well within 3 hours the cramps were gone and I had no more restless leg syndrome. I was really shocked that iron worked so fast but it truly did. I take it to this day w/o fail even tho' I'm no longer a vegetarian. The reason I put cured in quotes was that my doctor says it's not cured but "managed". It really doesn't matter to me as long as I can sleep and have no cramps. Good luck to you.

~~~~~~~~~~~~~~~~~~~~~~~~~~~~~

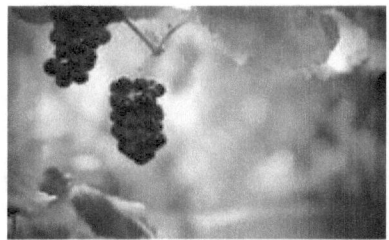

Weight Loss Experienced on Organic Foods

Posted on a "dieting" forum (this was just before being banished :/ :) . . . . one other who's experienced the same! . . . this was ignored however by the "diet gurus" :(

Thanks Crystbear!

Yes, I've experienced weight loss just by switching to organic meats and dairy. The growth hormones fed to chickens, cattle, pigs . . . but are a huge problem for our bodies . . . . adding tenacious fat-clinging calories. I feel sorry for all the children who balloon out just from eating normally and drinking milk loaded with these hormones.

~~~~~~~~~~~~~~~~~~~~~~~~~~~~

Digestion, Fibromyalgia and one other who went Organic . . . digestion

You can't feel good on all that medication.

I've been suffering for years with digestive issues and fibromyalgia. So much so I went back to school at The Institute for Integrative Nutrition and became a health counselor.

After a great summer i started having more and more sensitivities to foods. And I'm not talking about processed foods. I'm talking about real whole home cooked foods. Everything seemed to bother me. I am now listening to what MY body needs which is a very simple easy to digest whole organic foods so that my body has time to heal and adjust to my age and lifestyle. Healing is a journey, a lifestyle into healthier living.

Coming off of the medication is only the beginning.

~~~~~~~~~~~~~~~~~~~~~~~~~~~~

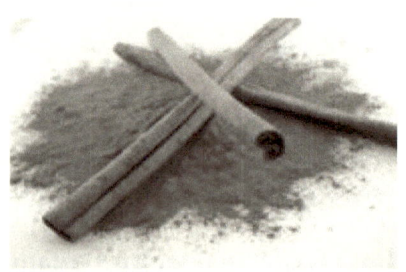

Cinnamon for arthritis/fibromyalgia relief

This is interesting, someone spoke of how his arthritis/fibromyalgia has been helped by taking 3 capsules of cinnamon at bedtime, and his pain has subsided . . .

Arthritis relief too simple to believe.

Wouldn't have tried this unless I'd seen it print. Cinnamon . . . that's all. My arthritis/fibromyalgia/RSD, whatever you want to call it, means I move around like a crab for a couple of hrs in the am, but taking 3 1000mg caps (available @ Sam's, or make your own) eliminates 80%+ of this most of the time.

Should have mentioned . . . .

I take it @ bed time.

~~~~~~~~~~~~~~~~~~~~~~~~~~

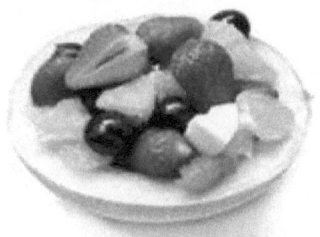

Vitamin C and Allergy

Actual experience *********** cat allergy & vitamin C

A few months ago, my neighbor and I visited a friend in a nearby building. While two of us played chess, my neighbor was playing with the cat. Shortly after that, I noticed him constantly wiping his eyes with a tissue. After several minutes I realized something was unusually wrong when he continued to wipe his eyes every few seconds. His eyes were puffy, and watering relentlessly.

He was considering taking an antihistamine. I said don't do anything for 8 minutes. I ran home and grabbed a bottle of ester-C powder, a measuring spoon, and a timer.

Upon returning, I gave him 1/2 teaspoon ester-C (1000 mg) in a few ounces of water, and started the timer. I told him in 5 minutes he may or may not notice an improvement, and in 10 minutes he should begin to feel better.

After 5 minutes I asked if he was getting any better. He thought maybe, but wasn't sure. After 10 minutes [total] I asked again. Although not completely symptom free, he was definitely beginning to feel relief, and was observably no longer in distress. At 20 minutes there was no question that an improvement had occurred. I suggested he take another 1000 mg for complete relief, but [like a sissy] he declined. The next time we went to that friends house, he took vitamin C first.

I don't know to what extent auto-suggestion can help, but would suggest you try vitamin C. Ester-C is [in my opinion] the very best, and it's acid neutralized.

~~~~~~~~~~~~~~~~~~~~~~~~~~~

Vitamin C and Asthma

Since I heard here about vitamin C for asthma and have been taking it I have had less asthma attacks. I was really in bad shape with asthma til I started the C. I now take about 2000 mg a day and doing much better.

My question: How long have you been taking it?

"A few days, its really helping and we have allergies to our cat which it helps. I'm going to take around 5 grams a day and see how I feel. I've just been taking 1 a day.

I am taking 2 grams a day, 1 gram in the morning and 1 gram in the evening, which is 1000 mg each.

I also drink alkaline water all day, which helps to keep the vitamin C in my tissues rather than being flushed out in the urine . . ."

~~~~~~~~~~~~~~~~~~~~~~~~~~~~

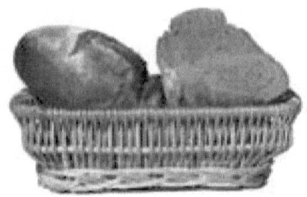

Cholesterol Lowered Naturally crystbear, I'm with you
I couldn't take statin drugs, so I did the whole grain breads and cereals, I dropped my LDL over 150 points and raised my HDL by over 50 points.

Just personal experience

~~~~~~~~~~~~~~~~~~~~~~~~~~

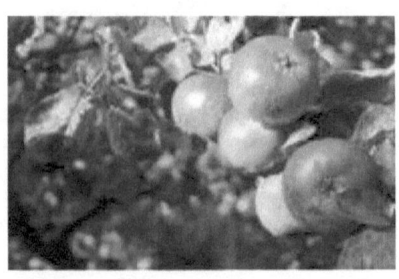

Hemorrhoids and Apple Cider Vinegar?? Yep wow . . . thankyou! crystbear! (2 days later after mentioning yeast infection and how apple cider vinegar may help) **as soon as you said yeast infection, i knew it . . . that's what it felt like originally coming on, but i knew they were hemmroids and i didn't put the two together. i immediately applied acv directly and while it burned it was nothing compared to the burning insatible itch . . . anyways . . . i just keep applying . . . i'm so happy i think i can handle this w/o a doctor. :) "physician heal thyself" . . . i've also started to drink acv . . . it's something i've wanted to have in my diet anyways . . . also just going forward with as raw and fresh as possible . . . peace***

~~~~~~~~~~~~~~~~~~~~~~~~~~~

Apple cider Vinegar and Eczema . . .
Another poster brought this one to my attention regarding ACV and one's eczema . . .

Breakthrough: I have struggled with eczema my entire life. I have been prescribed so many pills and ointments. Tried so much stuff. Nothing helped.

I finally found a cure. Well, not a cure, but something that alleviates it greatly.

Apple cider vinegar

I dilute it with water, rub it on my skin, leave it on for 15 minutes, shower it out. My skin feels so calm. Not itchy at all.

I know it works because I tried it for five days. The three days I used it, my skin was so calm. I stopped using it for two days and I started getting itchy again the second day. Then I used it yesterday and my skin calmed down again.

I'm so happy I could cry. This has been a lifelong search for a cure. I've taken medication. I've used ointments. I've changed my diet. Changed my soaps, etc.

Now I know how normal people feel. :)

~~~~~~~~~~~~~~~~~~~~~~~~~~~

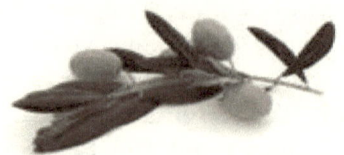

Kidney Stones, Olive Oil and Lemon Juice

Not one, not two, but three "anecdotal" testimonies for this same remedy! However it is duly noted that conventionals say it is impossible to happen . . . hmmm :)

I read this first on earthclinic.com posted it to help someone, and one responded who actually tried it and acknowledged how it worked for him also! And then a third posted the *same* post to help someone else because it helper her son too! . . .

Try olive-oil and lemon juice followed-by—a glass of water . . .

"I have suffered intermittently from kidney stones for nearly 9 years. One was so bad I had to have surgery to remove it. Later, my grandmother was hospitalized with a kidney stone and told me about a home remedy given to her by a nurse and believe me, this really works! Mix 2 oz of olive oil and 2 oz of lemon juice, drink it straight down and follow with a large glass of water at the first sign of stone pain. The stone(s) will pass within 24 hours. I have eliminated at least 8 stones with this remedy and have not gone back to the urologist since I started taking this." And one responded:

"I did this last month with a 7 mm stone and the <—> urologist was a little upset that it dissolved the stone. He was going to do a very expensive procedure on me that would have been both invasive and painful." Then one other referred to it and posted it again today having it help her son too! . . .

"I read this on here last year when my son was dealing with kidney stones and it worked. Sure can't hurt. Sorry you're going through all this, my son said it was pure hell."

I think we're on to something here! I hope many more will be helped also with this "impossible" remedy:)

~~~~~~~~~~~~~~~~~~~~~~~~~~~~

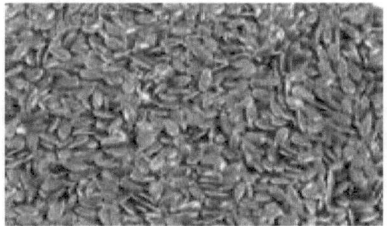

Cottage Cheese, Flax Seed Oil, and Stage 3 Lung Cancer

My son (now the total organic health nut) showed me this one on youtube . . . who responded to one of his own posts . . .

"**My dad was diagnosed with stage 3 lung cancer about a year ago . . . He was 79 at the time and did not want any form of treatment . . . I started him on the cottage cheese and flax oil and some of the cancer has shrunk and has not spread . . . He is stable with no coughing, good appetite and has been getting good reports . . . He does this 2x per day and so far so good . . . We feel it's better than nothing and the doctor just shakes his head in awe when he sees him . . . We thank God for this treatment.**"

~~~~~~~~~~~~~~~~~~~~~~~~~~~~~~

From A.I.M . . . .

Hi, we don't know one another but I loved your blog. I have been studying natural health and herbs for 30 years and it sickens me just to know how much the public is not informed when it comes to the food they eat, and all the conflicting health information . . . I find your site straight forward and informative which is refreshing in today's world/environment.

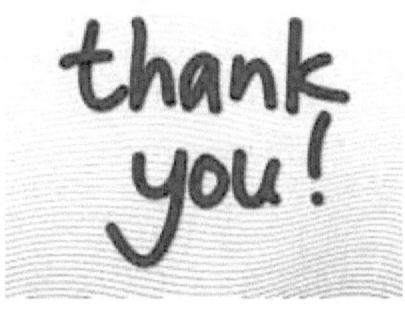

Note: please heed some warnings if you're taking other medications, and always consult your physician first.

Information and accounts written here and throughout this book are for entertainment and not intended as a substitute for the advice provided by your physician or other healthcare or holistic professional. You should not use the information for diagnosing or treating a health problem or disease, or prescribing any medication or other treatment.

Please remember: Vitamin supplements may have allergy affects in rare cases. Some vitamin supplements may also conflict with any medications you are taking as well. Always consult with your doctor before taking them.

_____

==

Rustic's Healthy Recipes :)

How you can get healthy, be happy and *save money* is by making your own organic healthy food! So, here are some recipes to help you. I hope you enjoy them as we do:

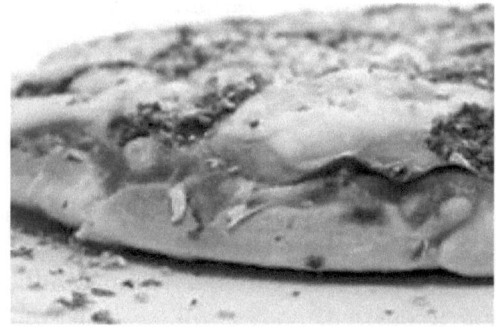

Rustic's "Healthy" Organic Pizza Recipe

3-4 cups whole wheat or regular unbleached . . . or mix of both . . . organic flour
2 pkgs. dry yeast
1 1/4 cup very warm water (110 degree)
2 tablespoons organic evoo
1 tablespoon organic honey
1 table spoon organic sugar
1 teaspoon sea salt

In mixer bowl, combine hot water, honey and evoo and dry yeast, let stand 5 minutes for yeast to activate. Add 3 cups flour, then add 1sp. sea salt. Mix with dough hook 10 minutes . . . add flour as needed to keep from sticking to bowl. Take out, knead 12 times. Place in oiled bowl, cover, and let rise for 1/2 hour. Take out on floured surface and cut in half (makes 2 pizzas).

My Basic Organic Topping (This is as close to my grandma's from sicily as I could get)

Mix together the first 5 ingredients:

1 can organic chopped tomatoes (I remember she used whole tomatoes and squished them by hand)
2 cloves of organic garlic chopped
1/2 teaspoon organic dried red pepper flakes
1 teaspoon organic dried oregano
3 Tablespoons organic evoo
2 packages shredded organic mozzarella
Organic Pepper and Sea Salt as desired

Topping suggestions: Grated parmesan, pineapple chunks, green and red pepper strips, chopped basil, parsley, bacon (browned and crumbled), and extra chopped garlic if desired.

Roll out 1 of the halves of dough to round pizza pan size. (wrap other in plastic wrap and keep in refrigerator if using later or you can freeze) Spread 1/2 of sauce mixture on one, sprinkle organic mozzarella, grated parmesan cheese and oregano if desired, and sprinkle with evoo. Add any of the Topping Suggestions you wish at this point as well.

Bake on bottom rack of 425 degree oven for about 15 minutes (check after 12 minutes).

*   *   *

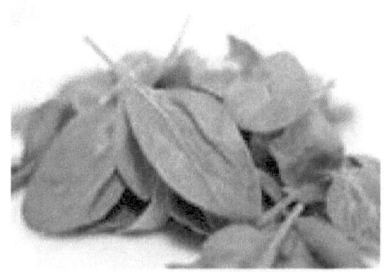

Rustic's Healthy Quinoa Salad with Baby Spinach, Cranberries and Avocado

2 Cups organic Quinoa
3 1/2 cups filtered water
Bring to boil and simmer 15 minutes or so

In a medium bowl combine the following and let stand:

2 cups organic baby spinach
1 cup organic dried cranberries (because I love dried cranberries in salads and stuffings, you can add more or less)
1 Avocado diced (safe list)
1/2 onion chopped small (safe list)
Lemon juice (about 2 organic lemons)
EVOO
Sea salt and organic black pepper to taste

Put cooked quinoa in a Large salad bowl and let cool. When quinoa is cooled, add in the above salad mixture.

*   *   *

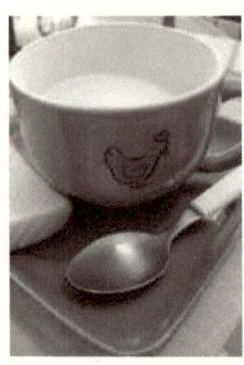

Rustic's Healthy Homemade Chicken Soup

Large pot of (filtered) water
1 or 2 leftover whole roasted free range chicken w/bones
Boil and simmer for about an hour
Let cool then remove chicken from bones and put in a bowl.
In chicken stock put in:
5 or 6 organic carrots (I just make 2 or 3 inch long cuts)
4 or 5 stalks of organic celery sliced (same)
1 onion, chopped or sliced
3 or 4 cloves of organic garlic, sliced
2 or 3 cut in strips organic green or red or yellow peppers (1/2 a bag of frozen organic from my market)
1 or 2 handful of organic baby spinach sea salt and black pepper red pepper flakes to taste
1 organic lemon

Put carrots, celery, onion, garlic, pepper strips with sea salt, black pepper and red pepper flakes in stock, and simmer until vegetables tender, about 1/2 hour.

In the mean time, shred all cooled chicken from bones, then add back into pot to heat up.

Squeeze lemon juice into soup or into individual bowls.

Serve with grated parmesan and/or hot sauce if desired.

*   *   *

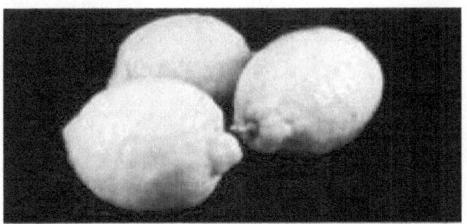

Rustic's Healthy Lemon Wild Shrimp with Vegetables

1 lb wild caught (not farm raised) shrimp (shells and veins removed)
1 bag frozen organic asparagus (if you have fresh (safe list) by all means use them)
1/2 bag frozen organic pepper strips (same if they are organic)
4 organic garlic cloves chopped
1/2 cup white wine
1 heaping tsp organic corn starch (found online) (no gmos)
2 or 3 squeezed organic lemons
1 tablespoon organic sugar filtered water (about a cup or so)
EVOO
Sea Salt and Pepper to taste

Heat large non-stick (green) fry pan with EVOO
Saute asparagus and peppers in EVOO with S&P to taste, and put in large bowl
Deglaze with white wine, add chopped garlic and shrimp, cook a few minutes
Mix corn starch in about 1/2 to 1 cup water with the lemon juice and sugar, add to shrimp and stir until heated through and shrimp are pink.
Pour this over vegetables.
Serve with brown rice if desired.

*   *   *

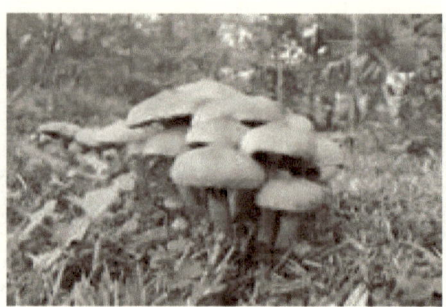

Rustic's Stuffed (safe list) Mushrooms

2 portabella mushrooms   Sea salt & org. black pepper
1/2 bag of frozen spinach defrosted   Parmesan cheese
1/2 bag of organic mozzarella   2 minced garlic cloves
1/2 cup dried bread crumbs   EVOO

Cut off stems and scrape off gills. Saute each mushroom in evoo 3 or 4 minutes. mix spinach, mozzarella, dried breadcrumbs, minced garlic, (or garlic powder) salt and pepper to taste in bowl.
Stuff each mushroom with mixture.
Grate parmesan cheese on top of each
Sprinkle a little evoo on top.

Bake 350o 15-20 minutes

*   *   *

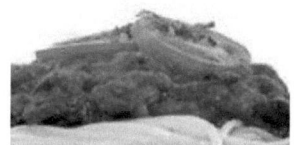

Rustic's Organic "Meatless balls" and Spaghetti

I don't always have grass fed meat, so I tried this "plant based" meatless meatball and it was pretty close to my original:

For the "meatless" balls:

1 can organic kidney beans (drained and rinsed)
1/3 loaf wholegrain organic italian loaf
1 organic egg
1/4 cup parmesan

3 org. garlic cloves
1/4 onion chopped (safe list)
1/4 cup chopped org. parsley

Put all in food processor and mix till thick consistency (looks like mixed chop meat).

Roll into meatballs and brown in evoo on all sides.

Put in sauce to cook another 10-15 minutes.

For the Sauce

2 cloves organic garlic minced
1/2 onion chopped
EVOO
organic hot pepper flakes
1/2 teaspoon organic dried oregano
Sea salt and organic black pepper to taste

1/2 cup red wine
1 lg. can org. crush tomatoes
1 small can org. tomato paste
1/2 cup water
1/4 cup chopped org. parsley

Saute onions, then garlic in Evoo, add red pepper flakes, oregano, sea salt and black pepper (to taste). Add redwine. Stir in tomato paste and water. Add large can of crushed tomatoes. Cook for a few minutes, then stir in parsley.

Organic Whole wheat spaghetti

Cook spaghetti in water as directed.

Cook sauce.

Brown meatless balls.

Add into sauce.

Serve over spaghetti with grated parmesan if desired.

*   *   *

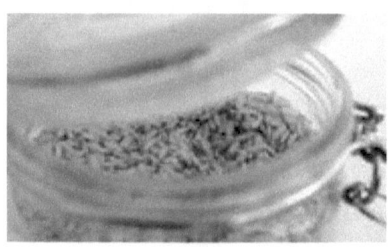

Rustic's Organic Brown Rice & Egg Bowl

An easy and low cost go-to recipe that you can adjust any way you like . . .

2 cups organic brown rice	Organic Evoo
4 1/2 cups water (filtered)	1/2 cup white wine (or chicken stock)
organic coconut oil or organic butter	2-3 handfuls of org. baby spinach
2 large garlic cloves chopped	4-6 organic eggs
1 onion chopped	Sea Salt and Org Black Pepper to taste

Cook brown rice in 4-5 cups water with coconut oil (or butter) as directed . . . usually 45 minutes.

Saute chopped onion and garlic (I chop them both in food processor together) in evoo a few minutes

Deglaze pan with white wine (optional) or water or chicken stock if you like

Add to this:

2-3 handfuls of organic baby spinach til wilted . . .

while spinach is wilting . . . whisk

4-6 organic eggs—whisk with fork in small bowl . . . then add to onion/garlic/wine/spinach mixture in pan . . . stir with wooden spoon till cooked through . . . spoon in cooked brown rice . . . . mix together . . . and as Chef Ramsey would say . . . "done!"

Can splash in some organic low salt soy sauce, or hot sauce if you like

*　　*　　*

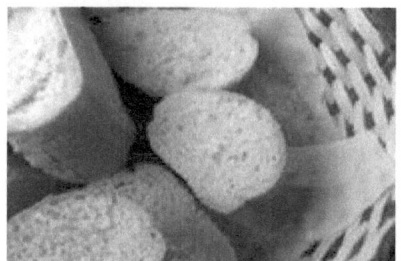

Rustic's Organic Bread Recipe

If you have an automatic bread machine, you can simply use organic ingredients! But if you don't, I think this recipe is just about as easy . . .

1 pkt organic yeast
1 cup warm (110 degree) filtered water
3 cups organic flour
2 tbs organic evoo or coconut oil
1 1/2 tsp of sea salt or himalayan salt

In mixer bowl put dry yeast, 1 cup of flour and 1 cup of warm water. Stir and let stand for 40 minutes.

Add to mixer bowl 2 cups of flour, oil, sugar and salt, with dough hook on mixer, knead on low for about 20 minutes. Take out and knead by hand 12 times, then place in oiled bowl. Let rise in warm place for 2 more hours.

Knead a few times by hand, form into loaf, and put in oiled loaf pan. Let rise another hour in warm place.

Bake 350 degrees for 1 hour. Cool 5 minutes and remove.

* * *

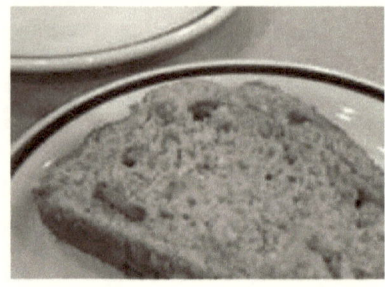

I now like to incorporate coconut whenever I can, and so I did with this recipe as well:

Rustic's Healthy :) Banana Coconut Nut Bread

3 ripe organic bananas
2 organic eggs beaten
2 cups organic flour
3/4 cup organic sugar
1 teaspoon sea salt
1 teaspoon baking soda
1/2 teaspoon organic vanilla extract
1/2 cup chopped walnuts
1/2 cup unsweetened coconut

In large bowl, mash bananas, add eggs and sugar and mix well (with fork). Add flour, sea salt and baking soda, mix with fork till blended well. Stir in vanilla, walnuts and coconut. Pour in greased loaf pan.

Bake 350 degrees oven 1 hour

Bananas have two times as many carbohydrates as an apple, five times as much Vitamin A and iron and three times as much phosphorus. In addition, bananas are also rich in potassium and natural sugars.

* * *

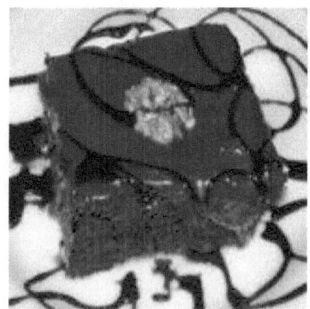

Rustic's Organic Dark Chocolate Cake

INGREDIENTS

For the chocolate cake:

1/2 cup organic unsweetened cocoa
hot water and organic milk
1 cup unbleached organic flour
1/2 tsp sea salt
1 tsp baking soda

4 tbsp softened organic coconut oil
1 cup organic sugar
1 organic egg yoke
1 tsp organic vanilla extract

PREPARATION:

For the chocolate cake:
Preheat oven to 350 degrees.

In a 1 cup measure, put cocoa powder. Add enough hot water for the powder to dissolve with a fork, and then fill the rest of the cup up with milk.

Combine flour, salt, and baking soda, mixing well with a fork.

Beat softened coconut oil and sugar, add egg yolk, beating for one minute. Stir in vanilla and combine everything.

Mix for one minute. Turn batter into a greased (with coconut oil) 8 x 8 pan.

Bake for about 35 minutes or until cake tests done. Place on a cooling rack.

For a chocolate icing:

You can simply dust organic powdered sugar on it if you wish (I found online). I also make a simple gnache (organic dark chocolate and heavy cream with a little organic sugar and vanilla with 1 tablespoon instant coffee granules) melted together and poured on top. Serve with unsweetened whipped cream if you wish.

*　　*　　*

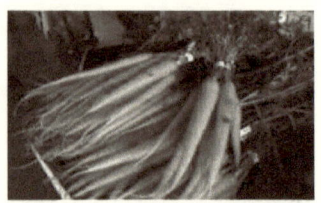

Rustic's "Healthy" Organic Carrot Pineapple Cake

butter and flour a 9x13 inch pan
2 cups all-purpose organic flour
2 teaspoons baking soda
1 teaspoon baking powder
1 teaspoon sea salt
2 teaspoons organic ground cinnamon
1 3/4 cups organic sugar

1 cup melted coconut oil (anti-fungal)
3 organic eggs (Vit D, omega 3)
1 tsp organic vanilla
2 cups organic shredded carrots (beta carotene)
1 cup organic unsweetened flaked coconut
1 cup chopped organic walnuts (omega 3s)
1 cup fresh pineapple "crushed" in processor

For icing . . .

1 (8 ounce) package organic cream cheese
1/4 cup organic butter, softened
2 cups organic confectioners' sugar (found online)

Directions

Preheat oven to 350 degrees F

Mix flour, baking soda, baking powder, salt and cinnamon. Make a well in the center and add sugar, oil, eggs and vanilla. Mix with wooden spoon until smooth. Stir in carrots, coconut, walnuts and pineapple.

Pour into prepared 9x13 inch pan. Bake at 350 degrees for about 45 minutes. The center will sink a little. Allow to cool.

To make the frosting: Cream the butter and cream cheese until smooth. Add the confectioners sugar and beat until creamy. I sprinkle with unsweetened coconut or chopped walnuts.

Carrots are rich in Vitamins A, C, K and potassium. Health benefits of the carrot include the following: Prevention of Heart Disease: Carrots on a regular basis can reduce cholesterol. Prevention of Cancer: Beta-carotene consumption reduces risk of cancer notably lung cancer. Fiber rich carrots reduce colon cancer. Rich in Vitamin A carrots improve eyesight.

*   *   *

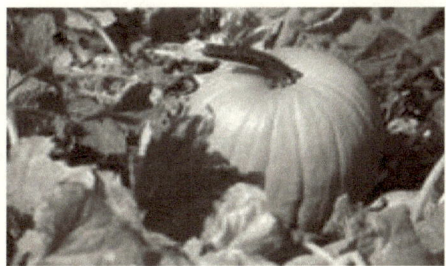

I found these two recipes last fall, and converted them to healthy organic using coconut oil:

Rustic's converted Organic Pumpkin Bars with Cream Cheese Frosting

Ingredients:

Bars

4 organic eggs
1 2/3 cups organic sugar
1 cup melted organic coconut oil
1 can (15 ounces) organic pumpkin (found online)
2 cups organic all-purpose flour

2 tsp baking powder
2 tsp organic ground cinnamon
1 tsp sea salt
1 tsp baking soda

Directions:

Preheat oven to 350 degrees and grease a 9x13 baking dish.
Mix the eggs, sugar, oil and pumpkin with a mixer until light and fluffy.
Pour flour, powder, cinnamon, salt and baking soda into another bowl and mix.
Pour flour mixture into pumpkin mixture and mix until incorporated and smooth.
Pour the batter into the baking dish and level out the batter.
Bake for 30 minutes or until a toothpick inserted in the center comes out clean.
Remove from the oven and allow to cool before removing from the dish or frosting.

Frosting

1 package (8 ounces) organic cream cheese, softened
1/2 cup (1 stick) organic butter, softened

3-4 cups organic confectioners' sugar
1-2 teaspoons organic vanilla extract

Frost the bars when they have cooled. Combine cream cheese and butter in a bowl and mix until smooth. Add the sugar slowly until you reach the desired consistency. Stir in the vanilla.

—

Rustic's Converted Organic Pumpkin Bread

3 c. organic flour	1 tsp sea salt
2 c. organic sugar	1/2 tsp baking powder
2 tsp. baking soda	15 oz of organic pumpkin (found online)
1 tsp. organic cinnamon	2/3 cup melted coconut oil (cooled)
1 tsp. nutmeg	3 organic eggs lightly beaten

Preheat oven to 350 degrees. Grease 2 9 x 5 loaf pans. Stir dry ingredients in large bowl, then wet ingredients. Pour half full in pans. Bake 1 hour.

Pumpkin flesh gets its orange color from beta-carotene, an antioxidant called carotenoids. Beta-carotene may help reduce cell damage in the body and improve immune function. It may also reduce your chances of developing chronic diseases such as heart disease. Rich in Vitamin A is also beneficial for the eyes.

*   *   *

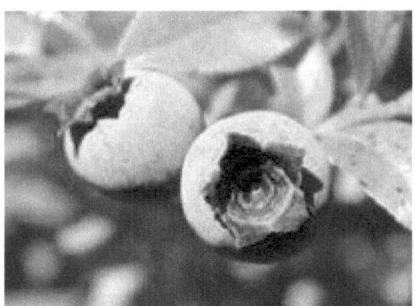

Rustic's Organic Coconut Pancakes with Wild Blueberry syrup

For Coconut Pancakes:

1 1/2 cups org a/p or ww flour (or mix of both)
1 Tbs org sugar
1/8 to 1/4 cup org coconut flakes
1 tsp. sea salt or himalayan salt
1 1/2 tsp baking powder (without aluminum)
3 Tbsp. org coconut oil
1 1/4 cups org milk
1 org egg

In bowl mix the first 5 ingredients. In measuring cup mix the milk, egg and coconut oil, then add into dry ingredients and stir (I used a fork) till completely incorporated.

I used a 1/4 cup measure cup to drop each pancake into melted coconut oil. Cook on medium to low heat til done.

For Wild Blueberry Syrup

1 bag of organic frozen wild blueberries
A tbsp or so of organic corn syrup (found online)
1 tbsp organic sugar or organic stevia
splash of water

Combine and simmer all in small saucepan until syrupy consistency. Spoon over coconut pancakes.

"Superfood" blueberries help with memory loss, cardiovascular health, blood sugar/diabetes, and arthritis! Enjoy :)

*　　*　　*

Rustic's Organic Dark Chocolate Banana treats

2 organic bananas cut into round slices (about 1/2 inch or desired thickness)
3 1/2 oz organic 85% dark chocolate
1/4 cup organic unsalted peanut butter
1 tablespoon organic corn syrup (I found online)
1/2 teaspoon organic vanilla
organic shredded unsweetened coconut

Put chocolate, peanut butter, corn syrup and vanilla in heavy pot to melt (carefully on low) or in bowl over simmering water.

Remove, place in bowl and let cool a little

Dip banana slices in melted chocolate mixture, place on wax paper on a tray sprinkle coconut on top of each and freeze (about 20 minutes or so), and have a "rustic" *healthy* treat! :)

Just fyi! The above recipes are *not* for "weight loss" *per se* (before all you "diet gurus" rip them apart *calorie by calorie*:) They are *simply organic* healthy recipes I have and use, some more often than others . . . depending on the *"mood swing"* I'm in :)) heh

* * *

This book was written for informational and/or entertainment purposes only, and not intended as a substitute for the advice provided by your physician or other healthcare or holistic professional. You should not use the information for diagnosing or treating a health problem or disease, or prescribing any medication or other treatment. The above recipes may be evaluated by your doctor or nutritionist (if you are on a special diet) to see if they are appropriate for your own healthy condition.

Wishing you good health and happiness :) God bless rustichealthy